Medicine in Sports Training and Coaching

Medicine and Sport Science

Vol. 35

Series Editors
M. Hebbelinck, Brussels
R.J. Shephard, Toronto, Ont.

Founder and Editor from 1969 to 1984
E. Jokl, Lexington, Ky.

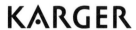

KARGER

Basel · Freiburg · Paris · London · New York · New Delhi · Singapore · Tokyo · Sydney

Medicine in Sports Training and Coaching

Volume Editors
J. Karvonen, Helsinki
P.W.R. Lemon, Kent, Ohio
I. Iliev, Sofia

68 figures and 18 tables, 1992

KARGER

Basel · Freiburg · Paris · London · New York · New Delhi · Singapore · Tokyo · Sydney

Medicine and Sport Science

Published on behalf of the
International Council of Sport Science and Physical Education

Library of Congress Cataloging-in-Publication Data
Medicine in sports training and coaching/volume editors, J. Karvonen, P.W.R. Lemon, I. Iliev.
(Medicine and sport science; vol. 35) "Published on behalf of the International Council of Sport
Science and Physical Education." – –T.p. verso.
Includes bibliographical references and index.
1. Sports medicine. I. Karvonen, Juha. II. Lemon, P.W.R. (Peter W.R.) III. Iliev, I.
(Iltho) IV. International Council of Sport Science and Physical Education. V. Series
[DNLM: 1. Physical Education and Training.]
ISBN 3–8055–5517–2 (alk. paper)

Drug Dosage
The authors and the publisher have exerted every effort to ensure that drug selection and dosage
set forth in this text are in accord with current recommendations and practice at the time of
publication. However, in view of ongoing research, changes in government regulations, and the
constant flow of information relating to drug therapy and drug reactions, the reader is urged to
check the package insert for each drug for any change in indications and dosage and for added
warnings and precautions. This is particularly important when the recommended agent is a new
and/or infrequently employed drug.

© Copyright 1992 by S. Karger AG, P.O. Box, CH-4009 Basel (Switzerland)
Printed in Switzerland on acid-free paper by Thür AG Offsetdruck, Pratteln
ISBN 3–8055–5517–2

Contents

Contents

Dedicated to Pawlinka, Mary Ellen and Anna-Liisa

Preface

Until recently, sports medicine and coaching have been more or less separate disciplines with little overlap. As a result, there is a dearth of literature with a balance treatise of medicine in coaching, i.e. the common ground between medicine and coaching. Moreover, the existing meagre interdisciplinary literature has been aimed almost exclusively at the scientific community. In the present work, specialists in medicine and coaching outline ten of the major medical issues in elite sport. The intention was not to produce a technical handbook of coaching but to provide medical guidelines for coaches and health professionals involved in elite sport.

In addition, 'Medicine in Sports Training and Coaching' gives a coherent review of the physiological, psychological and medical limits of physical performance. Exceeding these limits may lead to a state of overtraining, e.g., when the intensity and volume of training is increased too rapidly. Although the limits of individual physical performance are reached easily when the increase in training load is excessively rapid, these limits can be extended substantially by means of gradual adaptive training. Supportive evidence for this can be found in the development of top athletes over the past hundred years.

The contributors to 'Medicine in Sports Training and Coaching' feature renowned authorities from five different countries. In addition to scientific expertise, the contributors have a great deal of practical experience with elite athletes and coaches. As will be apparent from the table of contents, the various chapters not only deal with the medical evaluation of athletes, but also provide new insight into popular themes such as nutrition, heart rate monitoring, high-altitude training, and doping.

Finally, we would like to acknowledge Prof. M. Hebbelinck and Prof. R.J. Shephard, who were involved in this work on behalf of S. Karger AG, Basel.

March, 1992

Juha Karvonen, MD
Peter W.R. Lemon, PhD
Iltho Iliev, MD

Karvonen J, Lemon PWR, Iliev I (eds): Medicine in Sports Training and Coaching.
Med Sport Sci. Basel, Karger, 1992, vol 35, pp 1 21

Medical Management of Elite Athletes

Dieter Kabisch, Kleinmachnow, FRG

Contents

Introduction

Optimal health is a fundamental requirement for all athletes because it is necessary for the systematic long-term training required for top performance. Similarly, personal best performances are only possible if the athlete is healthy at the time of the competition.

Therefore, medical management should be directed towards measures that not only contribute to the development of optimal health and allow the completion of well-designed training programs but also help to identify and prevent health risks during the training process.

This can only be achieved with regular medical counselling and instruction of the athlete in matters of health. To be successful, medical management has to be integrated into the training program. This necessitates complete and mutual understanding among the athlete, the coach and the sports physician. The athlete must understand that the chosen medical measures are as important as any other component of training.

Medical management should be introduced early in an athletic career in order to help the athlete reach her/his true potential. Besides assessing health status, the sports physician must also assess the stage of physical development in relation to the specific demands of the athlete's event (early/late physical developer, estimation of final height, etc.). The purpose of medical assessment by the sports physician is to help the athlete and the coach ensure that:

(1) Health is maintained during the training process, or that possible changes in health status are recognized and treated in time.

(2) Physical development is evaluated during the training process, and that special biological characteristics as well as the potential performance

capacity are analyzed properly and given appropriate consideration in designing the training program.

(3) Medical opinion is part of the selection of talented young athletes for top-level training.

(4) Design of training programs is appropriate, paying special attention to connective and supportive tissues.

(5) Instructions are given concerning hygiene and preventive health-care.

(6) Important discoveries and insights of sports medicine are integrated into the coaches' education.

The *purpose* of medical evaluation by the sports physician should not only be to repair damage, but primarily to *prevent* it. To achieve that, medical measures have to be integrated into the training process (fig. 1).

Basic Physiological Factors

Biological Adaptation
Physical conditioning aims to improve existing physical abilities and skills in order to reach a higher performance level, whether it is in sports or

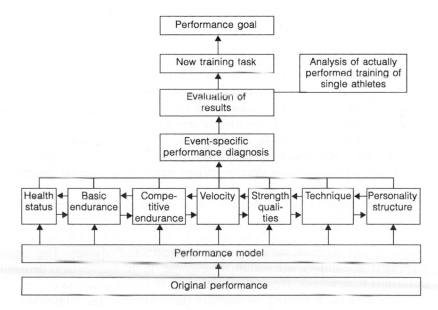

Fig. 1. Key components of the training process.

in everyday life. The potential for this lies in the fact that biological systems are able to react to external stimuli, to balance themselves accordingly, and – if the stimuli are repeated frequently – adapt to them.

Biological adaptation is the method the organism uses to respond to the demands it is subjected to. Adaptations occur as a result of the demands placed on the system and are predictable. Therefore, it can be stated that biological adaptations occur systematically.

Findings and insights concerning the ability of the human organism to adapt to physical exercise make up the biological foundations of training theory and methodology. Appropriate consideration and application of this knowledge is essential for an efficient training process (determining training loads). Otherwise performance or health will suffer.

This is where medical counselling and evaluations are needed and important both for the coach and the athlete.

Homeostasis, Heterostasis and Epigenetic Adaptation

Humans, as we know today, appeared about 40,000 years ago as a result of biological adaptation to natural and social environmental changes extending over thousands of years. This phenotype, i.e. the genetic program coded in the nuclei of each cell, can only be changed over many generations. As a result, the so-called *genetic adaptation* has no immediate significance in sports. No one can perform better than his genetic program allows. Inborn physical limits are of importance in many sports, and should be given appropriate consideration in the medical management of athletes.

More important in terms of designing training programs are those adaptational processes that are possible within the limits of the genetic system of each individual (*epigenetic adaptation*). The organism has a tendency to keep all organ systems in a state of balance (*homeostasis*), and, in case of disturbances (*heterostasis*), to normalize the situation as soon as possible. The organism can be characterized as a thermodynamically open, self-regulating, multistable system, which adapts in order to maintain a stable internal environment despite various external or internal influences [1].

One example of such a disturbance of physical function occurs with the increased muscular activity of sports performance. It results in an immediate increase in metabolic demands, which again leads to further reactions, such as increased heart rate and breathing frequency. The whole represents a complex adaptational response to a momentary demand disturbing homeostasis. Physical conditioning in sports is always connected with and directed towards a momentary disturbance of the homestasis.

When the demand (work load) ceases, adaptational reaction is decreased

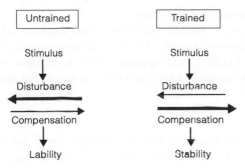

Fig. 2. Schematic depiction of the reaction by an untrained and a trained person to a defined stimulus.

(phase of restitution), heterostasis is converted again towards homeostasis, and the organism returns to its normal state of balance.

If the organism is repeatedly and at consistently shorter intervals subjected to increased exercise demands, it 'learns' to maintain the normal functional values longer in balance, and to restore deviations more quickly. This kind of adaptation allows better control of demands and leads to an increased performance capacity. At the same time, it protects break down of the system itself (fig. 2).

Thus, the organism learns to cope with constant or repeated demands. This takes place via systematic changes of function (functional adaptation) or of organ structure (morphologic adaptation). Hypertrophy of the skeletal muscle (increased cell size) as a response to strength training is an example of such a structural change. This results in increased contraction power and strength.

General and specific features of adaptation, objective assessment of the adaptational status, or of duration and extent of the restoration phase in single organ systems require constant cooperation between the sports physician and the coach in order to ensure a sensible and effective training program.

It is particularly important to pay attention to the close relationship among the different levels of adaptation. Israel [2] has described three different levels:

Specific (event-specific) adaptations which occur as a response to the training methods used for a particular event. These occur primarily in the muscle groups used for the specific movements, and in their regulation and maintenance systems. Adaptational changes occur mainly in the neuromuscular area, and these are apparent in the motor capacity of skeletal muscles.

General (Performance-Specific) Adaptation

General adaptation refers to the internal functional capacity of the organism in relation to performance-specific demands. It serves to maintain vital functions during heavy loading, and applies mainly to organs, functions and regulatory systems controlled by the autonomous nerve system and hormones.

Cross-Adaptation

Cross-adaptation refers to the fact that a stimulus does not only provoke adaptation in the systems directly influenced by it, but that adaptational changes also occur in other areas of the organism. These changes can be either positive or negative in nature.

Positive cross-adaptation occurs when there is an adaptational gain. Negative cross-adaptation leads to an adaptational loss. In the case of positive cross-adaptation, adaptational processes contribute jointly to improved performance, whereas with negative cross-adaptation competition develops, resulting in a decreased performance.

Adaptation is always dependent on the training load. For that reason, changes will be lost and the organism will return to the former state if the stimulus (work load) discontinues. Thus, adaptational changes cannot be stored, but have to be induced over and over again. Acquired abilities begin to grow weaker as soon as they are not used regularly.

To sum up, the organism is not only ready to 'learn', but also to 'forget'. Every single training unit must therefore be constructed with the underlying biological principles in mind. Relevant questions as to sensible training programs can only be resolved with cooperation between the coach and the sports physician. Further, regular evaluation by a sports physician can reveal and perhaps prevent inappropriate loading, misadaptations and subsequent health disturbances.

Objectives of Medical Management in the Training Process

Depending on the event, development of an elite athlete may take from 5 to 8 years. This period of time can usually be divided into three phases, i.e.:

Basic training, which normally applies to children and youngsters between 10 and 14 years of age (however, in figure skating and gymnastics this may begin as early as 6–7 years of age). The training program consists of four to five 2-hour training sessions per week, and aims to teach general athletic foundations along with single event-specific elements. The essential goal is the systematic development of physical trainability and optimal

health so that the athlete can tolerate increased work loads at later stages
of the training process.

Build-up training helps enhance the development of young athletes to
the exercise and performance level of the elite performer. This involves
several training sessions per day, using rapidly increasing loads and highly
intensive training methods. This training phase is characterized by increasing individualization, striving for consistently better integration of all the
factors influencing the competitive performance.

Training for top performance is designed to lead the individual athlete
to the world-class level. It is constantly adjusted depending on the timing
of major competitions, highly individual and composed of a wide range of
exercises, applications and intensity levels. It requires complete command
of event-specific techniques and tactics, and is based on a stable health
status and maximal loadability.

Medical management by the sports physician is most efficient when the
measures are specifically adepted to the training phase. Every phase con-
centrates on different tasks and areas. On the basis of our own experience,
we suggest the following approach:

Basic Training
A medical evaluation should be performed at the beginning of the
training process, and thereafter every 6 months. This should guarantee
that:

(1) Only healthy, trainable children and youngsters are selected for
the training process.

(2) Health is maintained during the training process, or that changes
in health status are recognized before problems result.

(3) Physical development is evaluated during the training process, and
that special biological characteristics as well as the potential performance
capacity (early/late physical developers) are analyzed properly and given
appropriate consideration in designing the training program.

(4) Development of high general trainability is guaranteed, paying
special attention to connective and supportive tissues from the viewpoint of
sports medicine.

(5) Medical opinion is considered in the selection of talented athletes
with good development potential.

(6) Instructions are given concerning sportsmanlike life style.

(7) Important discoveries and insights of sports medicine are integrated into the education of coaches and physical instructors working with
youngsters. Finally, it is important to realize that the basic training phase
is by no means elite training on a smaller scale, and that the young athletes
are not miniature copies of world class athletes. On the contrary, age- and

developmental-specific features of children and youngsters must be given primary consideration.

Build-up Training

A weekly medical consultation by the sports physician is necessary to ensure:

(1) A constant up-to-date sports-medical diagnosis of health status and trainability.

(2) Adequate recovery is provided between intensive training units.

(3) Early recognition and treatment of health disturbances.

(4) Proper nutrition and sportsmanlike way of living.

(5) Exercise physiology principles are used in short-, middle- and long-term planning of the training process.

(6) Medical opinion is considered in the judgement of the expected performance potential of the athlete.

Training for Top Performances

Medical consultation is indicated daily. Besides continuation and intensification of follow-up procedures started in earlier phases, special attention should be paid to:

(1) Presence of medical service at single training units.

(2) General preparatory and rehabilitatory ('postparatory') measures in order to ensure high trainability and rapid, complete recovery.

(3) Prescription of specific sports-medical measures during the pre-competition period, on the competition day and after the competition (nutrition, fluid balance, vitamins, physical therapy, etc.).

(4) Medical treatment in case of illness or injury.

(5) Instructions concerning the transition period after ending top sports.

A systematic outline of medical measures found to be necessary in different events can be especially effective. Medical activity (measures, their extent and frequency) needs to be incorporated into all training periods. Each sports association should have a sports physician on its Board, and he/she in turn should establish a medical commission, which outlines the forms of activity needed at different levels. The commission would also be responsible for its implementation with the help of local sports physicians, and, last but not least, for close cooperation with coaches in order to ensure integration of all necessary medical services into the training programs of elite athletes.

The primary goal for medical management is effective prevention of health problems instead of secondary treatment of disturbances or injuries. Therefore, prospective planning, organization and management are essential.

Inevitably, a management process of this kind creates a permanent long-term, very personal relationship among the athlete, coach and physician. If medical consultation is limited to the treatment of injured or sick athletes and if different physicians are used, it is difficult to establish the confidential relationship necessary for the athlete to attain her/his true potential.

Appropriate medical management is *prospective* medical activity covering the complete range of factors influencing the athlete and his/her performance. It can only occur in cooperation with the athlete and coach.

Medical Evaluation

Medical evaluation in sports medicine can be divided into the following areas:

(1) Examinations concerning physical characteristics necessary for the specific event.

(2) Basic assessment of health status and stage of physical development.

(3) Diagnostic tests concerning trainability and other event-specific matters.

These examinations are all event-specific and, therefore, only give general guidelines, common to all events, can be given.

Initial Examination

Sports History. Initial entrance into sports, event, first competitive training and achievements in sports (best results and placings).

Medical Anamnesis. Anthropometric measures according to Wutscherk [3]: body height; body weight; shoulder width; pelvic width; right forearm circumference (male); right thigh circumference (female); measurement of active body mass (lean body mass); biological age; assessment of final body height.

Clinical examinations: General health status, nutritional status, examination of skin and visible mucous membranes (icterus, cyanosis, edema, exanthema).

Head examination: Mobility, sensitivity to pressure/percussion and headache.

Eyes: Sharpness of vision, reaction to light, convergence, rough examination of visual field, bulbar mobility.

Ears: Auditory sense, otoscopy.

Balance organs: Romberg test, Fukuda-stepping test.

Mouth: Mucous membrane, dentition, gingiva.

Cervical organs: Tonsils, pharynx, thyroid gland, lymph glands.

Thoracic organs: Thorax (symmetry), respiration; lung (lung lines, percussion sound, respiratory sounds).

Heart (size, percussion finding, action, sounds): Pulse, blood pressure.

Abdominal organs: Omentum, liver, spleen, kidneys, hernial 'gates', pathological resistances.

Spine: Examination of general posture (examination with reference to the vertical or when standing on two spring scales), assessment of shoulder and pelvis status, and of leg length.

Orientational Examination of General Mobility (Forward Bend, Backward Bend, Side Bend). Functional diagnostics according to the principles of physical therapy.

Extremities: Mobility, tonus and nutritional status of the musculature; assessment of articular contours and ligaments; examination as to functional or reflectory disturbances of the muscles.

Central nervous system: Patellary reflex, Achilles reflex, Babinski reflex, pupillary reflex, coordinative tests (finger-nose test, knee-heel test).

Laboratory examinations; Cell count, blood sedimentation.

Urinalysis: Protein, glucose, sediments.

ECG: At rest, extremity electrodes I, II, III, aVR, aVL, aVF thoracic electrodes $V_1 - V_6$; immediately after exercise (30 squats in 30 s), extremity electrodes I–III; 3 min after exercise, extremity electrodes I–III.

X-ray examinations are performed according to a standard program. Further laboratory tests (e.g. liver enzymes) only if indicated on the basis of history and clinical findings. These may include blood group, sex chromatin, immunological status, dental examination, and orthopedic examination (if clinically indicated).

Special attention should be paid to following organ systems: Connective and supportive tissue (especially symptoms of weakness of connective tissue).

Nose and throat (especially predisposition to chronic inflammations).

Spine: note especially deviations in position or form of the spine, or constitutional hypermotility.

Extremities: axis deviations, deformities.

Muscle-ligament apparatus: disturbed motor-dynamic stereotypes, muscle coordination failures.

Special assessment criteria: functional status of the opto-vestibulospinal system; functional status of the spine and joints; assessment of arthromuscular balance.

Basic and Follow-up Examination

Intermediate Anamnesis

Anthropometric Data. Estimation of biological age and final body height once per year (until the 15th year of life).

Clinical examinations
(a) Laboratory examination:
   (1) Leukocytes, urinary status.
   (2) ECG: every second year (if not indicated according to inter-
       mediate anamnesis).
   (3) X-ray examinations according to a standard program.
(b) Special examinations:
   (1) Dental examinations (twice a year).
   (2) Orthopedic examination (every second year).
   (3) Gynecological examination (once a year after menarche).

Diagnostic Examinations on Current Trainability

Up-to-date diagnostics as to the trainability of an athlete is an essential task of sports medicine. It is, however, not easy, and differs according to the specific requirements of the event. Successful diagnostics is only possible with daily or at least twice weekly analysis of factors influencing performance.

In addition to the general aspects (clinical examinations, body weight, basic heart rate, etc.) up-to-date diagnostics deals with event-specific loading patterns and with the functional systems, organs and tissues which limit performance.

In most events, these controls include evaluations of:
(1) Connective and supportive tissues, especially spine, knee and other joints and tendons along with tendon-lubricating tissues and attachments.
(2) Organs of the cardiopulmonary system.
(3) Skin (hands, fingers, buttocks).
(4) Metabolism.

Can be accomplished practically by:
(1) Presence of medical experts at training sessions.
(2) Regular clinical evaluations by a sports physician.
(3) Event-specific performance diagnostics.
(4) Frequent evaluation of training programs.

Factors to be assessed continously: success of the training program; basic endurance; event specific endurance; velocity; strength endurance; maximal strength; event-specific techniques; sensomotor status; mental training; mobility; flexibility, etc.

Examinations of this kind are event-specific. Therefore, a more detailed description of them falls outside the scope of this book. Almost all endurance events use metabolic controls in order to analyze the performance structure (morphologic and functional requirements and quantitative or qualitative energy demands during competition). This is because adaptation of the muscle to contraction requirements is reflected in the metabolism. It is up to the sports physician to see that the role of aerobic, alactic and lactic energy production in each event is considered in the design of the training program. The same applies to the diagnostics of the cardiovascular system (functional diagnostics) and of selected strength parameters.

Maintaining and Improving Health Status and Physical Performance Capacity in the Training Process

A methodologically correct training program is the key for maintaining health and preventing connective and supportive tissue injury in top sports, as well as at earlier stages of an athletic career. One of the essential factors in this respect, is an evaluation of the dynamics of recovery after exercise and the adaptation processes in single organ systems [4].

Examples of postexercise recovery times (depends on degree of depletion as well as diet during recovery): circulatory system – a few minutes; carbohydrate metabolism – approximately 6 h; connective tissue – 8–24 h.

For this reason, findings of sports medicine and recent research are of essential importance for planning of training programs. Special attention must be paid to the adaptation of connective and supportive tissues because of their extremely long recovery times.

Tests of muscular function are very important and informative with respect to the functional status and susceptibility to injury of supportive and motor apparatuses. They should be performed every 3 months because antagonist and synergist muscles must always be in balance relative to each other.

This can be reached when the following five principles are observed:
(1) Individual Loading
Several factors should be considered including:
    (a) Biological age (e.g. childhood, adolescence).
    (b) Training years.
    (c) Constitutional factors (e.g. weakness of connective tissue).
    (d) Inborn abnormalities of connective and supportive tissues (e.g. abnormal menisci).
    (e) Momentary status of the connective tissue (e.g. 'minor injuries' microtraumas).
    (f) General health status.

Caution is indicated with continous loading after minor injuries or too early postoperative loading, as they may cause irreversible damages.

(2) Systematic increase of loads

Slow adaptation of connective tissue requires progressive increases in training load over a long time period. Rapid progression or large increments should be avoided.

(3) Load and recovery

Important factors include:

    (a) Prophylactic spine extension after exercises which stress the spine.

    (b) Distribution of exercises which stress the connective tissues into several training units per day.

    (c) Use of several short training sessions instead of one long session because this is more favorable with respect to the supportive and motor apparatus.

    (d) Avoid extensive loading of connective tissue and complicated movements especially when muscles are fatigued.

(4) Sufficient warm-up

Methodologically appropriate warm-up is beneficial for:

    (a) Musculature: loosening-up of musculature; increased muscular elasticity; improved stretching ability.

    (b) Connective tissue: improved nutritional supply, and hence improved loadability.

    (c) Neuromuscular system: improved coordination and reaction ability.

As a result injury incidence can be minimized.

(5) Versatile strength training

Versatile strength training plays an important role in the prevention of joint injuries.

Fourteen Theses in Sports Medicine

Sports medicine of the former German Democratic Republic (GDR) has summarized these principles into the following 14 theses (5):

Thesis 1: Increased Loadability of the Supportive and Locomotion System Is an Elementary Requirement for Improved Sports Performances

Progressive improvement of the physical performance in sports requires command of ever-growing loads in training and competition. In most events, this is not possible without a parallel improvement of the loadability of the supportive and locomotion system (SLS). The most vulnerable points differ from event to event; damages of joint cartilage and tendon attachments are perhaps most typical.

Recommendations for training;

Screen and examine ways to improve the loadability of the SLS in your event. This applies to all levels of training (basic, building-up and top-level).

Be very precise when increasing loads to be sure that they do not exceed the athlete's capacity and are in accordance with his/her biological development.

Change the training load, if there are symptoms from the event-specific vulnerable points of the SLS.

Improve your training documentation in order to register the loadability of the SLS.

Thesis 2: Arthromuscular Imbalance during Basic or Build-up Training Interferes with Development of the Event-Specific Movement Coordination

It has been demonstrated that heavy training loads (especially event-specific loading) can lead to an above-average incidence of arthromuscular imbalances even during basic and early stages of build-up training. This can interfere with the development of event-specific movement stereotypes. Moreover, arthromuscular imbalances reduce the loadability of joints.

Recommendations for training:

Use regular stretching and strength exercises during all phases of training.

Add to the volume of stretch and strength programs in the same proportion as the amount of intensive training increases.

Use stretch and strength programs as subunits of training session before and after intensive loads, and as autonomous training units (specific SLS training).

Thesis 3: Distinct Arthromuscular Imbalances Reduce the Loadability of the SLS

Distinct arthromuscular imbalances are one of the main reasons for reduced loadability of the SLS. They can lead to disturbances of motor stereotypes, accumulating overloads and, as a result, to damage or injury of the SLS.

Arthromuscular imbalances can be diagnosed and influenced by means of training methodology.

Recommendations for training:

Regular evaluations for shortened or weakened muscles (exercise-medical and sports methodological tests on muscular function).

Assessment of general physical training and of strength and stretch programs by means of muscular function tests (twice a year in basic training, every 3 months during building-up and top-level training).

Use the results of exercise-medical and sports methodological tests on muscular function, along with norm controls and tests as reference data in training documentation.

Complete the documentation with findings of kinesiologic tests (posture, joint mobility, muscular strength).

Employ regular methodological correction of demonstrated muscular imbalances through the use of versatile, general physical exercise, stretch programs, strength programs and active relaxation.

Thesis 4: Rapid Load Increments and Technical Faults
May Lead to Overexertion of the SLS

Rapid increments in training load, maximal strength training with peaks affecting the joints, and technical faults due to muscular fatigue (in exercise series with many repetitions) can create a substantial stress on the supportive and locomotion system. It has been prepared for this by means of appropriate methodological measures.

Recommendations for training:

Include exercises which prepare the SLS for increasing loads into the training program.

Prepare the SLS for rapid load increments and high demands of the performance.

Use appropriate strength exercises to ensure that there is sufficient strength potential to maintain joint stability.

Use appropriate recovery periods so that the athlete can develop the appropriate technique (avoid technical faults).

Avoid prolonged training periods and high peak loads if there are signs of muscular or psychological fatigue.

Strive for joint agreement between the coach and sports physician concerning the form, suitability and timing of load increments and maximal loads.

Thesis 5: Rapid Growth in Height May Cause Temporary
Changes in General Loadability and Motor Coordination

During phases of accelerated growth (growth spurts at puberty), general loadability of the SLS, as well as the coordinative capacity may suffer a temporary loss. This refers especially to growth in height and loads to instability of the event-specific coordination in young athletes. As a result these athletes are biologically predisposed to overloading and injuries of the SLS.

Recommendations for training:

Modify the training pattern during growth bursts. Increase loading by means of versatile general physical exercises, concentrating on the training volume, stabilization of the changed motor coordination and re-establishing the arthromuscular balance.

Avoid high load impulses, maximal strength training and exercises requiring high muscular strain.

Thoroughly prepare the athlete for load increments and the altered external training conditions.

Thesis 6: The Supportive and Locomotion Apparatus Shows Longest Adaptation Time after Load Increments during Building-up Training

Progressive load increments are necessary in basic and building-up training. However, it must be understood that the supportive and locomotion apparatus needs the longest adaptation time of all organ systems. Consequent methodological prevention of overloading and injuries is an effective tool in increasing the loadability of the SLS. Prophylactic measures must refer to the whole range of training from general design to details (weak points of the SLS, especially knee and ankle joints). Exercises putting a special strain on the SLS must be known and controlled appropriately.

Recommendations for training:

Ensure a favorable, stable development of physical factors to the athletes to endure the training load. This can be accomplished by using versatile basic physical exercises.

Follow the principle of load and recovery in designing the training regime and weekly rhythm. Ensure psychophysical recovery and active relaxation.

Develop your athletes' command of the basic technical and coordinative skills to avoid training overload and injuries of the SLS. Check for proper landing techniques or economy of the running movement, use falling exercises, etc.

Protect knee and ankle joints (arthromuscular balance) by means of active and passive (knee protectors, bandages, etc.) measures.

Thesis 7: The Supportive and Locomotion Apparatus Needs Systematic Preparation for Complex Load Increments

Long-term improvement of sports performance occurs through systematic complex load increments from year to year, or from one training stage to the next. This should occur in a proper relation to the achieved loadability of the SLS (especially of joints as functional units) in order to ensure the effectiveness of the planned load design. The SLS is prepared for complex load increments bearing in mind the biological age and momentary loadability (general and event-specific performance capacity) of the athlete. The SLS needs continuous stabilization.

Recommendations for training:

To ensure adaptation of the SLS to higher loads, transitional training periods should be used

To avoid injuries or overloading (microtrauma) of the SLS, complex load increments should be used only when the biological age corresponds with the chronological age of the athlete.

For late physical developers, training programs need to be modified individually (more gradual load increments over longer time periods). Complex training program demands have to comply with the child's actual loadability.

Thesis 8: Special Training Using Maximal Intensity Must Be Prepared Properly and Followed by a Cool Down

Maximal efforts may lead to overloading and injuries, if not prepared properly, or if the musculature is fatigued. The principle of loading and recovery of the arthromuscular structures needs special attention in cases of arthromuscular imbalance, former injuries of the SLS, technical faults or high intensity demands. Recovery of the cartilage tissue takes considerably longer than recovery of the muscle tissue.

Recommendations for training:

Special training (especially during the precompetition period) requires systematic long-term preparation (improvement of general performance factors, year round technical training, etc.).

Careful organization of special training during meso- and microcyclic training can reduce overloads and drop-outs.

The principle of loading/recovery must be respected within a single training unit as well as within microcycles (warm-up, serial pauses, active compensatory exercises, relaxation exercises).

Arrange a minimum time interval between training units containing high intensity exercises or exercises with intensive shear or high muscle tension loads (in specific jump training 2–3 days).

Avoid technical training with high intensity exercises when the musculature is fatigued. Do it at reduced load intensity.

An acute fatigue of strained musculature should be treated clinically by a sports physician.

Thesis 9: Central Nervous Activation Promotes Motor Learning

Insufficient central nervous activation or training demands that exceed the actual activation level (demanding coordinative training of performance techniques) will result in a high incidence of failures in movement coordination. This increases the risk for overloading or injuries of the SLS. Training sessions with high technical and coordinative demands require a continuously high central nervous activation.

Recommendations for training:

Learning of motor skills and training with high technical and coordinative demands is most valuable at certain times within a day and week period. They are known in many investigations and this knowledge has to be used in the training design.

Always begin a training session with central nervous activation of the athletes by means of event-specific warming-up programs with duration at least 20–30 min.

Control the efficacy of the methods of central nervous activation using appropriate tests, like reaction time and tapping.

Thesis 10: Joints Are the Weak Points of the Arthromuscular System and Need Special Strengthening

Overstrain and injuries are most likely to occur in regions or parts that are not sufficiently prepared for high exercise demands. Joints are one of these 'weak points' of the SLS and frequently limit the exercise increments. Training intensity can be increased following strengthening of joint-stabilizing muscle groups and by paying special attention to the arthromuscular condition. Knees, ankles, lumbar spine, elbow and wrist are those joints that need special muscular stabilization because of the high pull and pressure strains they are predisposed to.

Recommendations for training:

Determine which joint structures are submitted to the highest load in your event (arthromuscular weakness), and make a note of that into your training diary.

Develop suitable exercise programs in order to increase the loadability of these weak points. These exercises can be completed either as specialized training or as a part of daily training or strength training.

Define and control exercise intensity and results of joint-stabilizing exercises in your event.

Use preparatory, joint-stabilizing exercise *before* maximal loads throughout the training year.

Thesis 11: The Position of Body Axes Can Be Maintained by Means of General Athletic Exercises

From the exercise-medical point of view, maintaining the positions of the axes (weight-bearing and rotational axes) of large joints (hip, knee, ankle) and of the spine is an essential requirement for optimal load increments. Axis deviations reduce loadability, especially of the knee joint. The weight-bearing axes of the body is determined in early childhood. Stabilization of the foot arch is based on the tension of tibial and fibular musculature. Regular, improperly compensated muscular fatigue can lead to loss of foot arch stability, especially in childhood.

Recommendations for training:

A harmonious development of the above-mentioned muscular 'loops' can be encouraged with the help of a bicycle or bicycle ergometer. The fatigue-resistance can be trained, especially gluteal muscle, lateral and medial leg extensor, anterior tibial muscle.

Better development of this muscular balance requires almost complete leg extension (see for appropriate adjustment of saddle height and pedal length).

By increasing the workload with bicycle or bicycle ergometer training, the above-mentioned muscular 'loop' can be strengthened and coordination improved, especially when the pedals have to be pulled upwards.

Thesis 12: Active Foot Strike Prevents Uncontrolled Joint Sprains

Uncontrolled foot strike as the end-phase of a performance creates an extremely high load on the feet, especially on the tendon and cartilage structures. Joint-stabilizing muscular function is therefore important, particularly at the beginning of the foot strike phase. Appropriate muscular pretension and coordination during foot strike is ensured by means of technical training of the landing process. This way, uncontrolled joint sprains can be reduced to a minimum.

Recommendations for training:

Correct foot strike techniques must be practised and continuously perfected from the basic training phase onwards.

An optimal foot strike technique strives for a long braking path, which enables a 'soft' landing.

The absorbance capacity of the foot is best utilized, if the load from the landing blow is directed towards the ball of the foot.

Thesis 13: Arthromuscular Balance of The Knee is of
Crucial Importance for The Loadability of The SLS

In most events the knee joint is the weakest point of the SLS. Systematic improvement of its loadability can be achieved with muscular strengthening programs improving the arthromuscular balance. Microtrauma of the knee joint should be prevented. Mechanical damage has to be reduced to a minimum, securing, however, an optimal perfusion of the knee joint area during loading. Therefore, knee pads are necessary in certain sports. Besides absorbing blows, they serve as warm-packs.

Recommendations for training:

Prophylactic use of knee pads should be obligatory in all events setting high loads on the knee joint (apparatus gymnastics, volley-ball, weight-lifting, track and field, jumps, duel events, hand-ball and soccer). This helps to secure undisturbed long-term development of the performance.

We recommend knee pads with the following characteristics: external foam-rubber layer (thickness 2–3 cm), reinforced seams of the foam-rubber layer, internal opening in the back of the knee, no back seam, rubber band reinforcement at the upper and at the bottom end.

In events like rowing, canoeing, cross-country skiing and biathlon modified knee pads ensure optimal blood perfusion of the knee joint.

Thesis 14: Optimal Loading and Recovery of the Spine Is the Most Efficient Prophylaxis against Lumbar Lordosis

Some exercises may (maximal strength, strength endurance, explosive strength training and specific jump training) squeeze the intervertebral discs and cause their flattening. This accentuates the physiological curvatures of the spine, especially the lumbar spine, and can lead to increased lumbar lordosis. There is a certain reduction of body height during the day, depending on loading and recovery of the spine. To avoid inappropriate loading, compression of the vertebral axis should be relieved regularly in the training program.

Recommendations for training:

Ensure stretching measures relieving the spine after heavy exercises, in order to avoid negative effects of loading.

Exercises that strain the spine must always be balanced with strain-relieving measures. These measures are to be planned separately, and documented in the training program.

Adult athletes need short strain-relieving exercises during the training sessions, as well as additional stretching, following each training period.

Children require a 60-min rest for the spine in the horizontal position after every second training session. Recovery in the sitting position (lunch) would strain the spine further.

The effects of spine-loading exercises, and strain-relieving measures can be assessed by measuring changes in body height.

Conclusion

Medical management should be introduced early in an athletic career in order to help the athlete reach his/her true potential. Besides assessing health status, the sports physician must also assess the stage of physical development in relation to the specific demands of the athlete's event (early/late physical developer, estimation of final fight, etc.). The purpose of medical evaluation by the sports physician should not only be to repair damage but primarily to prevent it. To achieve that medical measures have to be integrated into the training process. In training for top performances medical consultation is indicated daily. Besides continuation and intensification of follow-up procedures started in an earlier phase, special attention should be paid to the presence of a medical service even at single training events. Up-to-date diagnostics as to the trainability of an athlete is an essential task of sports medicine. It is, however, not easy, and differs according to the specific requirements of the events. Successful diagnostics is only possible with daily or at least twice weekly analysis of factors influencing performance.

References

1   Israel S: In: Sportmedizinische Grundlagen der Körpererziehung und des sportlichen Trainings. Leipzig, Barth, 1987, pp 17–23.
2   Israel S: Grundprinzipien der bewegungsbedingten körperlichen Adaptationen. Körpererziehung 1985;35:293–300.
3   Wutscherk H: Die Anthropometrie in der Praxis des Kreissportarztes. Berlin, Sportmedizinischer Dienst, 1983, pp 33–35.
4   Berthold F, Brenke H, Dietrich L: Empfehlungen zur Vermeidung von Schäden am Binde- und Stützgewebe. Berlin, Sportmedizinischer Dienst, 1980, pp 6–22.
5   Neumann G: Zur Sicherung der Belastbarkeit des Stütz- und Bewegungssystems (SBS). Sportverlag, 1987, pp 6–15.

Dr. Dieter Kabisch, Im Tal 15a, D-O-1532 Kleinmachnow (FRG)

Karvonen J, Lemon PWR, Iliev I (eds): Medicine in Sports Training and Coaching.
Med. Sport. Sci. Basel, Karger, 1992, vol 35, pp 22–48

Drugs and Sports[1]

Emmanuel P. Gachev

Department of Biochemistry, National Academy of Sports, Doping Control Laboratory,
Research Centre of Sports, Sofia, Bulgaria

Contents

[1] These data are based on drug informations available by 1991.

Introduction

Are drugs applicable in sports? Yes, they are, both as medicines and, unfortunately, as doping agents. Drugs used as *medicines* are substances of various origin prescribed by doctors for medical purposes (prevention or treatment of diseases) within very strictly defined conditions of use (dose, duration, mode of administration, etc.). Thus, they can have beneficial or no effect at all, yet every measure is taken against possible health risks. When drugs are taken by athletes (in high doses, for a long time, etc.) with the purpose of improving sport performance despite the possible health risks, we speak of *doping*. Consequently, the same drug or drug preparation can both be a medicine or a doping agent, depending on the purposes and modes of its use. Such a distinction may be insufficient in itself to avoid confusion and eventual misuse, therefore it will be extended and specified later. What should be remembered is that athletes cannot use a number of banned drugs during the period of training or before competition. Allowed drugs are available with the presence of medical indications and, in some particular cases, the ways they can be used are also indicated. These are the reasons which make it necessary to draw a clear cut line between allowed medicines and banned drugs, i.e. doping. This is very important because a seemingly innocent drug preparation (e.g. one intended to treat a common cold or cough) may contain forbidden components. Its use will inevitably lead to a disqualification of a totally unaware athlete and may result in additional severe sanctions. Another more important reason why this problem shall be discussed in the following text is the health damage which may result from the use of doping. Very few athletes clearly and fully realize the nature and the gravity of this damage. It is sometimes associated with long-term or lifetime disability, infertility in the family and even death.

Now that pharmaceutical companies are manufacturing a large number of drug preparations with names which are not always directly informative of their composition, any self-treatment can present enormous health hazards. Moreover, regrettable though it is, there are still coaches and sports specialists who are not far from the thought of giving athletes drugs in order to increase their performance. Moreover, such substances are available on the black market. Hence, the only recommendation to be made is that athletes should not take drugs unless a physician or a pharmacist can guarantee that those drugs are free of doping agents.

The Doping Issue

Doping in the Past and Now

Various drinks and magic rituals have been used since antiquity to enhance a competitor's performance. Doping, in the modern sense of the term, seems to have been first used as a means of gaining victory (and profit) at the horseraces in England where big money was bet. Some of the participants in a swimming contest in Amsterdam 1865 are reputed to have used doping. This appears to be the first documented case with athletes. With the rapid advance of pharmaceutical industry, markets were gradually supplied with a growing choice of drugs which could, as some athletes still believe, ensure the victory. In his article 'The pill that can kill sports' Neal Wilkinson commented so about the Games in Melbourne 1956: 'This craze for pills was most shocking at the recent Olympic games. In Olympic village, the atheletes' rooms looked like small drug stores. Vials, bottles and pill boxes lined the shelves.' At the following Olympic Games in Rome, 1960, a Danish cyclist died in competition after the use of doping. Thus, the doping issue could no longer be discussed in the narrow terms of fair play only, but that it also concerned the health of the athletes. The actual campaign against doping could not yet begin, though. Imposed bans were often violated for the lack of objective and reliable methods of doping control. It was only in the late 1960s that the German chemist Manfred Donike, together with engineers of Hewlett-Packard, improved the nitrogen-sensitive detector of gas chromatographs. This opened possibilities for detection and confirmation of doping agents in samples of athletes' urine. On that basis Donike and his team of assistants carried out the first large-scale doping analysis at the Munich 1972 Olympics. 2,097 urine samples were tested and 7 athletes were disqualified. At the following Olympic games, in the summer of 1976 in Montreal, testing for anabolic steroids was started by the newly developed methods of mass-spectrometric analysis: 8 athletes were disqualified. Doping control techniques were improved to such an extent that at the Pan-American Games in Caracas, 1983, many athletes left to avoid testing. Of those who remained 19 were disqualified [1].

As will be shown further in the text, today the analytical and technical problems have been drastically minimized to the point where it is almost impossible to avoid detection.

Definitions of Doping

Once a given concept is defined in different ways this can only mean that there is no agreement on the principle underlying the definition. In other words, the concept is defined from different points of view. A group of definitions states that doping harms health and is, therefore, forbidden. According to other definitions doping is only an attempt at unfair play. These differences have made Sir Arthur Porrit, President of the British Association of Sports Medicine admit that 'to define doping is, if not impossible, at best extremely difficult, and yet every one who takes part in competitive sport or who administers it knows exactly what it means' [2].

The difficulties Sir Arthur refers to are obvious yet we can doubt that the problem is indeed so clear for 'everyone who takes part in competitive sport'. It must be recalled that the number of banned substances exceeds 240 [3]. Bearing this in mind in 1990 the International Olympic Committee (IOC) again defined doping as 'the use of prohibited substances and of prohibited methods'. Which are the prohibited substances and methods of doping? Doping substances are grouped in 6 pharmacological classes (i.e. the grouping is based on their effects in the body, rather than on their chemical structure). These are: stimulants, narcotics, anabolics, beta-blockers, diuretics and peptide hormones. Blood transfusion and urine manipulation are banned methods. Thus, the IOC Medical Commission obviously defines doping on the basis of lists of doping substances belonging to one of the mentioned classes. The lists of doping substances are open. They will automatically include all compounds of a specified type (i.e. having similar effects) that could be developed or used in the future. For this reason the lists under question are incomplete and open – they end with the words 'and related compounds'.

Some Words on Drugs: Relations between Drugs and the Body
There are different *routes* by which a drug can enter the body. Most drugs are administered by *mouth*. The process of their passing through the gut wall into the bloodstream is called *absorption*. This process is, by its duration and completeness, an essential factor determining the effect of a drug. The effect will be more potent if absorption takes minutes instead of hours, and if it is full and not partial. Many drugs are *injected*, under the skin, into a muscle, or directly into the blood-stream (into a vein). Injections are made when a rapid and potent effect is expected, especially when the same drugs taken by mouth are absorbed slowly or poorly. Some drugs are administered by *inhalation* (breathing into the lungs). An example is the inhalation of aerosols for asthma, or the smoking of marihuana (cannabis). The skin and the mucous membranes are also permeable to drugs. Various ointments, some of them containing banned substances, may be *rubbed* into or *applied* topically onto the skin; the nasal mucous membrane is a common route for a number of banned stimulants, among them cocaine.

Different drugs have different *distribution* patterns in the body. In principle, once in the blood stream a drug goes to the cells of the organ where its major effect is exerted. Thus, stimulants and narcotics interact predominantly with the cells of the central nervous system. Most drugs, sooner or later, follow a common pathway and go to the liver and kidneys. Their molecules are subject to chemical alterations which are generally termed *metabolism*. The altered products are *metabolites* of the parent drug.

The processes of transformation are localized mostly in the liver and this is the reason why the organ can so frequently be damaged by some groups of drugs. Another aspect of metabolism is that it determines the potency and the duration of the effect. Clearly, if in the course of metabolism a drug compound undergoes chemical changes and is transformed into a metabolite it will lose its biological effect. If the transformation is rapid and full then the expected useful effect will be short-lived. There are some exceptions, however, which make the actual picture rather complicated. It turns out that at times the metabolites, rather than the parent compounds, have therapeutic effects. At other times metabolites have more or less pronounced toxic effects in the body. Moreover, when a drug is metabolized rather slowly or when its elimination is slow, a new administered dose will sum together with the preceding dose. In this way a *cumulation* of the drug will result in several days which may be dangerous to health.

Most drugs leave the body partly unchanged and partly as metabolites. This is due to the role of the kidneys which excrete unnecessary products of blood into the urine. This process is called *excretion*. Drug excretion is very well known to chemists working in doping control laboratories. They know very well when a compound will appear in the urine after administration and as what metabolites.

The quantity of administered drug, i.e. its *dose*, is very important for its effect. Dosage depends on the mass of the body.

Many doping compounds are toxic when administered in rather high doses. Overdosage results either from ignorance or from the desire to achieve a stronger effect in a shorter time. A common, although absolutely erroneous, principle according to which 'more means better' is in action here. In fact, it must be well understood that many drugs with positive effects in lower doses can be toxic in higher doses. This rule is so valid that even substances considered as useful to health, such as vitamins, in higher doses lead to intoxication (hypervitaminosis) which in some cases may be lethal.

It should also be remembered that there exists an *individual degree of tolerance* to drugs. Thus, some individuals may react with *hypersensitivity* to some drugs. This phenomenon may be inborn or acquired, after single or repeated use of the same drug.

Simultaneous administration of several different drugs may also lead to poisoning because of *incompatibility*. All drugs causing such reactions should be immediately withdrawn.

Habituation to a drug is another unpleasant phenomenon. It can have different consequences. First, because of *resistance* the dose may have to be constantly increased. Second, it may lead to *drug dependence* because of addiction to a drug with all ensuing results.

Problems of Drug Nomenclature

Besides its precise chemical name every substance used as medicine has another, shorter name by which it is better known. Knowing only this latter name may not be enough, though, for two reasons. First, different companies manufacture the same drug under different proprietory (trade) names. Secondly, a drug is very often used as an ingredient of different combinations for different purposes. Naturally, names are so different that sometimes even an experienced specialist can hardly guess the actual composition. Very similar or misleadingly close names may be given to quite different substances or combinations, while the same substance may appear under different names. An impressive examples of the latter is the incomplete list of ephedrine-containing drug preparations, comprising more than 70 names. Most of these, moreover, are well known and widely used for common cold, flu, asthma, etc., and many of them are available over-the-counter, without prescription.

All this gives a clear idea of the dangers faced by an athlete using drugs even for purposes other than influencing sport performance. He may administer a doping agent unintentionally and be punished for that as the IOC Medical Commission will not accept explanations or justifications related to an incidental illness (common cold, etc.). Therefore, an athlete should always consult a physician or a pharmacist whenever he is taking a drug preparation and check for the absence of doping agents in it. This is not to mean that an athlete is given a less-favored treatment for his complaints. Efficient medicines free of banned substances are at an athlete's disposal in any case of ailment (cold, pains, asthmatic attack, inflammatory diseases, injuries, etc.).

Doping compounds are classified by the IOC Medical Commission in six classes, as mentioned above (stimulants, narcotics, anabolic steroids, beta-blockers, diuretics, and peptide hormones and analogues). In addition, there are some drugs whose use is subject to certain restrictions. Corticosteroid hormones and local anaesthetics are among the latter.

Stimulants

The function of muscles and many other organs are controlled by the nervous system. Hence, drugs which activate the central nervous system, e.g. cerebrum, brain stem, spinal cord, can exert an active influence on muscles and other vital organs, such as heart and lungs which are important for overall exercise capacity. Such compounds are generally termed stimulants, although they are divided into several groups with rather different characteristics.

An example of the more important groups will be reviewed in the following text. The first place is taken by the group having *amphetamine* as its major representative. Amphetamine is a potent central nervous system stimulant. It belongs to the psychomotor stimulants. It produces stimulation, increased activity and alertness, lifts up the mood by a feeling of wakefulness and strength, increases both the mental and physical performance and diminishes or delays fatigue. Arterial blood pressure is raised, pulse rate is accelerated, and bronchial muscles are relaxed causing a feeling of easier breathing. The stimulating effect lasts for 2–7 h and is often followed by tiredness, lassitude and headache. This is the reason for repeated administration of amphetamine which, in its turn, gradually leads to addiction. The real danger comes from the possible fatal depletion of the metabolic reserves of the cells. This is observed in the case of heavy physical loads, and is believed to have caused the death (on the track during the Summer Olympic Games in Rome 1960) of a Danish cyclist. The well-known and widely used *caffeine* also belongs to the group of psychostimulants. This alkaloid is found in tea leaves and in coffee and cola beans. It is rapidly absorbed through the intestines and produces a stimulating effect within 20–30 min which continues for 4–5 h and is most potent during the first hour [4]. Caffeine dilates the blood vessels of the brain, the heart and the skeletal muscles. Thus, it increases both the mental and physical working capacity. High doses of it, however, can cause insomnia, restlessness, headache, dizziness and sometimes convulsions. Detection of stimulants in urine, even in the smallest traces, is a reason for anti-doping sanctions. Caffeine is the exception: because coffee, tea, coca-cola, etc., are widely consumed. Therefore, the appearance of caffeine in low concentrations (below 12 mg/l) is not considered as doping. When more than one tablet of caffeine-containing drugs (see examples below) are taken, or when caffeine is injected, its concentration in the urine rapidly rises above the critical level and leads to antidoping sanctions.

Cocaine is a potent, but ill-framed psychostimulant causing drug addiction and dependence. It is applied on the nasal mucous membrane as a white powder. It rapidly enters the bloodstream but does not produce an actual increase in physical performance. Its major effect lies in causing euphoria, an illusory feeling of well-being and superiority which is often manifested in aggressive behavior. Higher doses of it can cause death due to paralysis of breathing and of heart function.

Ephedrine is a representative of a whole group of compounds which undoubtedly has stimulating effects on the central nervous system. For this reason their use by athletes is also prohibited. What should especially be noted, however, is that these compounds possess many other valuable therapeutic effects and are, therefore, widely used as medicines. Thus, they are the basic components of drug preparations against asthma for they relax the muscles of the bronchi. Allergic diseases of the respiratory pathways (rhinitis, sinusitis, bronchitis) are also treated with preparations of the ephedrine group. Finally, because the latter compounds suppress the appetite, they are used in a large number of slimming preparations in combination with vitamins and often seem innocent. Nevertheless, the IOC Medical Commission will immediately act accordingly to the detection of even negligible traces of compounds of the ephedrine type in an athlete's urine. For this reason a rather extensive, and yet incomplete, list is presented below of medicines and drug preparations belonging to this doping group. The list is to give an idea of the dangers threatening an athlete whenever he uses drugs, even for medical purposes, unless a physician or a chemist have checked beforehand that they do not contain doping substances.

Strychnine is also a stimulant, mainly of spinal cord function. It enhances the keenness of perception. Muscle performance is increased but not very significantly. Strychnine is eliminated slowly from the body and repeated use may lead to toxic accumulation. The latter, as well as the administration of high single doses, may cause very painful muscle cramps and in more severe cases death, because of paralysis of the central nervous system.

So far the lists prepared by the IOC Medical Commission contain over 80 banned stimulants. They are available for sale both as individual preparations and in combination with other compounds in drugs intended for various purposes. Their actual number exceeds several hundred and, obviously, an exhaustive presentation of them will go beyond the scope of this article. Athletes must be reminded again that the final and competent decision of whether a drug contains banned substances lies with the physician or the pharmacist and that self-administration can be extremely dangerous.

Finally, cases are to be mentioned, such as common cold, flu, asthmatic attack, etc., when an athlete has to use some drugs for treatment. A tentative list of drugs and drug preparations permitted and recommended by the IOC Medical Commission in such cases is presented below.

Narcotics

Narcotics, ore more precisely *narcotic analgesics*, are drugs chiefly intended to relieve or eliminate pain. Everyone knows that injuries, burns, inflammations, tumors, spasms, colics, etc., are often accompanied by severe pain and are medical indications for the use of narcotic analgesics. The problem actually has two sides. The first is that pain is a biological signal of failure threatening the organism and should not be suppressed until its causes are found or, as in the case of sports, eliminated. The other is purely medical: by itself very severe pain can have harmful consequences such as abrupt fall of blood pressure, loss of consciousness, etc., which should not be allowed.

Morphine, a plant alkaloid of opium, is one of the earliest means discovered long ago and used even today to treat and relieve pain. There are many other drugs which very closely resemble the structure and effects of morphine.

Morphine is valued as a medicine for two chief effects: potent relief of pain and suppression of the cough center. In addition, it produces *euphoria* (elated, happy mood regardless of reality). After the effect of morphine has faded euphoria is replaced by depression or intolerable mental discomfort. This is often the reason for turning to a new, higher dose because of developing tolerance and dependence, known as morphinism. Dependence on morphine is both psychic and physical. When the drug use is discontinued the following symptoms of *withdrawal* are observed: sweating, accelerated and irregular pulse (tachycardia and arrhythmia), drop in blood pressure and even epileptiform convulsions.

Morphine also has a potent cough suppressant effect and was earlier used in antitussive combinations.

Morphine suppresses the centre of breathing leading to slower breathing rate and respiratory depression which can cause death by asphyxiation (*asphyxia*) in case of overdosage. Morphine also increases the tone of bronchial muscles and can produce severe asthmatic attacks.

The other preparations of the morphine group possess the same effects expressed to varying extents. Thus, *codeine* (methylmorphine) has a 5–6 times weaker analgesic effect, produces almost no respiratory depression and the resulting euphoria and risk of dependence are much less. It has identical antitussive effects as morphine. *Dionine* (ethylmorphine) has an even stronger cough suppressant effect. For this reason dionine and codeine have replaced morphine in the antitussive combinations.

When and why would athletes take narcotic analgesics? Perhaps the most important reason is that training and competition efforts are often accompanied by unpleasant sensations and pain. For example, repeated lifting of a heavy bar-bell, for hours on end, is accompanied by pains coming from the critically loaded muscles, tendons and joints. Some athletes cannot achieve record weights without analgesics. This is connected with many dangers. The masking of pain, i.e. of the biological signal of stress or failure, such as the utmost load on the body, can result in ruptured tendons and muscles and dislocated joints. In a more general case the metabolic reserves can be fatally depleted because of unrealistic assessment of the proper potential and state at the moment. Excitement verging on aggressiveness can make up for the feeling of tiredness and fear in front of a stronger opponent. Such behavior is common after administration of *heroin* (diacetylmorphine). Clearly, there are legitimate reasons why an athlete might use narcotic analgesics. However, the latter can lead to drug addiction which is incompatible not only with sports but with the ancient principle of a sound mind in a sound body.

Apart from what has been described so far there may be cases of undeliberate administration of narcotic analgesics by athletes. This may occur during treatment for common cold or bronchitis and coughs. Drugs used to treat them very often contain codeine or ethylmorphine (dionine). It must be remembered that undeliberate administration of listed doping agents is unconditionally sanctioned. Of course, pains from injuries, migraine, toothache, colics, etc., need treatment and should be treated with non-narcotic analgesics. Examples of permitted drugs which can be used as pain relievers or cough suppressants are given in a separate list.

Anabolics

Anabolics or anabolic steroids are artificially made hormones. They were initially synthesized as chemical modifications of the main androgen, the male hormone testosterone. The stimulating effect of androgens on protein metabolism was established already in 1935 [5]. Testosterone was found to enhance the synthesis of the basic muscle contractile proteins, of blood proteins, etc. The direct use of this hormone, however, proved to be accompanied by desirable and sometimes even harmful effects of virilisation (appearance of male features in women) and suppression of the reproductive functions in both healthy women and in men (see below). This imposed a need to design artificially such chemical modifications of testosterone in which the androgenic or masculinizing effect was reduced while the effects on protein metabolism were preserved and enhanced. The new compounds were called anabolic steroids, anabolic hormones, or simply anabolics. In the early 1950s, athletes already started using them. With anabolics available, however, misuse of testosterone was not stopped. It went on for the entirely erroneous assumption that testosterone, as endogeneous product formed within the body would be more difficult to detect than exogenous (external or artificial) anabolic preparations. This is an illusion arising from ignorance of the capabilities of modern analytical equipment in control laboratories.

What are the effects of anabolic-androgenic steroids and how do they act in the body? These compounds easily penetrate the membranes that envelop both the cells and their nuclei. Once inside the nucleus they bind to the chromosomes, the cellular structures storing genetic information. (Genetic information is expressed through the synthesis of one or other type of proteins.) This is chiefly how the muscle, bone marrow and liver cells react. This results in increased amount of muscle proteins with concomitant increase of muscle size, lean body weight and total body mass [6–9]. Individual observations of increased muscle strength have been reported, but reports are rather controversial [10]. The positive effects of the use of anabolics lie chiefly in activating the processes of recovery after heavy and exhausting training, especially in power sports. Anabolics probably reduce the degradation of muscle proteins induced by training efforts and accelerate protein restoration and even supercompensation [8]. This is actually the main reason why they are used in sports. That effect, however, is achieved with rather high doses. Increased blood volume, and haemoglobin and plasma proteins content, were also observed. Whether these changes are accompanied by increased aerobic power is, however, debatable.

When administered for strictly medical purposes anabolic steroids are rather useful and effective. Thus, they speed up the healing of fractured bones, help the more rapid replenishment of lost blood after injuries and haemorrhage and reconvalescence after exhausting diseases.

What are the health risks of the use of anabolic steroids in sports? These substances, used in the negligibly low therapeutic doses (from 5 to 20 mg) in the course of few days only, have no influence on sports performance. Positive results, if ever, are achieved by means of considerably higher doses (almost incredible cases are reported of the use of 1,000 up to 1,500 mg daily), taken for months and even for years. Naturally, negative consequences of these high doses are possible. They comprise the following:

(a) Bone system: Premature calcification of the epiphyses (distal parts) of long bones. This stops growth in teenagers [11].

(b) Liver: Anabolics impair the functions and alter even the structure of this central metabolic organ. Elimination of toxic products through bile is impaired with resulting jaundice and toxic hepatitis. Cavities (cysts) full of blood form in the liver, their rupturing being fatal (peliosis hepatis). Occurrence of tumors is not a rare phenomenon; they may be benign, but also malignant [12, 13]. The hepatomas are chiefly induced by 17-alpha-alkylated derivatives (e.g. methyltestosterone, methandienone, methandriol, see list below). Health damage in the earlier stages is sometimes more difficult to diagnose and requires complicated equipment and methods (radioisotope and ultrasound scanning, computer tomography).

(c) Reproductive system: In both sexes anabolic steroids block the secretion of gonadotropins of the anterior pituitary, a gland in the basis of the brain. It produces hormones regulating the functions of other glands which, in turn, also produce different hormones. Gonadotropins, in particular, stimulate the functions of the gonads. Their blockage in men leads to impaired spermatogenesis and suppressed testosterone production by the testes, which gradually are atrophied [6, 14, 15]. Normal testicular function is restored, if ever, several months after the use of anabolics is discontinued. When the latter are administered in high doses, a part of them is converted in the liver into substances similar in effect to the female hormones. They, in turn, can cause gynecomasty in men, i.e. growth of the mammary glands [8]. In women, ovarian function is also blocked; menstruation stops, which naturally results in infertility. The external genital organs acquire masculine characteristics – the clitoris grows. If anabolics are applied at an earlier age then the body build also becomes of the masculine type: broader shoulders, facial hair growth and deepening of the voice are often irreversible results of anabolics use.

(d) Metabolism may be affected to a various extent [16–18]: Observations are reported of increased blood triglycerides and cholesterol, accompanied by decrease in the so called high-density alpha-lipoproteins. Observations in the author's laboratory indicate values of blood cholesterol reaching 10–11 mmol/l, instead of the normal 4–5 mmol/l in young athletes. This is quite unfavorable and in severe cases may predispose the individual to heart complications [19]. Carbohydrate metabolism is also affected.

Finally, anabolic steroids may also have psychological effects inducing aggressive behaviour. When their use is discontinued problems of withdrawal may occur because of developing dependence.

All these health risks give sufficient grounds for a strict ban on the use of anabolics in sports. The reader may refer to a detailed, yet unexhaustive, list of the most common anabolic substances and of the brand names of the drug preparations containing them. The list is presented at the end of the chapter.

Beta-Blockers

Cells in the body constantly exchange information by means of chemical signals, such as hormones and mediators. These substances exert their effects by binding to cells which possess specific structures for them, called *receptors*. For example, the hormone adrenaline appears in the bloodstream of an athlete who is excited about a forthcoming competition. This hormone, among other things, binds to receptors in the heart muscle and in the muscle cells of some blood vessels. As a result the athlete's pulse rate accelerates and blood pressure rises. This creates problems for everyone participating in a shooting contest: aiming will become more difficult because of more frequent and stronger oscillations of the hands and body.

Beta-blockers are drugs intended to block the functions of such receptors, called beta-adrenergic receptors. They suppress the excitability of the heart muscle, causing a slower pulse rate and lower blood pressure. For this reason they are applied with great success in medicine, but only after competent examination and careful supervision of the patient's health by a cardiologist. In some heart diseases (sino-atrial or atrio-ventricular block, etc.) beta-blockers can cause sudden death due to cardiac arrest. Severe asthmatic attacks are another possible complication. For these reasons, their use in sports is forbidden. There are other permitted drugs available to treat elevated blood pressure.

Recently, some beta-adrenergic receptor blocking agents, e.g. propranolol, have been used in strength and speed power sports to stimulate the release of growth hormone. Naturally, the use of beta-blockers for such purposes is also forbidden and shall be treated as doping.

Diuretics

About 6% of the body mass is water in the form of blood, lymph and intracellular fluid. Naturally this water contains many dissolved substances, first of all mineral (sodium, potassium and other) salts with precisely defined composition. The constancy of the composition of the body fluids is of vital importance. By forming urine the kidneys have a function to maintain the constant amount of water and salts in the body. Some diseases accompanied by edema (heart failure, liver failure, etc.) are part of the medical indications for therapeutic use of diuretics.

It follows that the use of diuretics by a healthy athlete can have negative consequences, disturbing the normal balance of water and salts in his body.

Athletes use diuretics mainly in two situations. One is associated with sports where athletes compete in strictly defined weight groups or categories. The rapid loss of weight (1–2 kg) will permit an athlete to compete in a lower weight category where he thinks he might have better chances for success. The other case is in itself an attempt at 'washing' out administered anabolics. Diuretics, taken for several consecutive days, are believed to minimize the chances of detecting anabolic steroids by doping control laboratories. The idea is theoretically naive, and the health risks of disturbing the normal water-electrolyte balance are quite real. Besides vomiting, weakness, dizziness, fall of blood pressure and muscle cramps the negative consequences may also include serious kidney and liver damage as, for example, with the frequent use of chlormerodrin or mersalyl.

Finally, in June 1987 the Cologne Laboratory of Prof. Donike found out that some athletes use *probenecid* to suppress the excretion of anabolics in urine. Probenecid is used in medicine to treat gout for it promotes the excretion of uric acid. This process interferes with the excretion of anabolics by suppressing it. Of course, the use of probenecid was immediately banned in sports.

It is clear from this review that there is absolutely no reason for a healthy athlete to use diuretics. A list of 11 most commonly used diuretics out of 41 available [3] is presented below.

Peptide Hormones and Their Analogs

Peptide hormones are *endogenous*, i.e. normally synthesized in the body, amino acid compounds. They play a very important role as chemical regulator signals to different organs, including the endocrine glands. They are either extracted from the organs and glands of human corpses or obtained synthetically by the methods of genetic engineering. Peptide hormones are administered parenterally by injection, because taken by mouth they are digested and become inactive. They are expensive and they are not always available. Important representatives of this group are somatotropin, gonadotropin, corticotropin and erythropoietin. They are detected in urine samples of athletes by means of radioimmunoassay.

Growth hormone (somatotropin, STH; Crescormon, Genotropin, Humatrope, Nanormon, Norditropin, etc.) is a potent anabolic hormone which controls growth. It is medically applied for overcoming retarded growth in children. It promotes the rapid healing of fractured bones and of various injuries. It seems, however, that growth hormone is increasingly used by athletes, either as a substitute of anabolic steroids or as their complement. It causes muscle hypertrophy and increased muscle size when injected in young healthy volunteers. But authors disagree as to whether muscle hypertrophy is indeed accompanied by increase in muscle strength [20, 21]. Non-medical use of the hormone is associated with different risks. Overdosage in prepubertal individuals will results in gigantism and reduced life expectancy. In postpubertal individuals high doses produce the disease acromegaly manifested with enlarged and deformed bones of the face, hands and feet. Diabetes mellitus, hypertension and early atherosclerosis are possible negative side effects. In addition, hormone preparations from pituitaries of corpse origin may transmit lethal viral diseases, such as Creutzfeldt-Jacob disease, AIDS, etc. Preparations on the black market are of unspecified quality, often faked and containing anabolic steroids instead of growth hormone. Use of propranolol (as mentioned earlier) to stimulate the endogenous production of growth hormone is, of course, forbidden.

Gonadotropin (pituitary or chorionic; available as Anteron, Choragon, Chorionic Gonadotropin, Gonabion, Gonadotrophon, Humegon, Kryptocur, Lutrelef, Pregonal, Predalon, Pregnesin, Pregnyl, Primogonyl, etc.). This peptide activates the male gonads and thus increases the endogenous testosterone production. Hence, the idea is to achieve a desired anabolic effect. From the point of view of anti-doping rules its use is analogous to that of anabolics (discussed above).

Erythropoietin is a peptide with hormonal action. Normally it is formed in the kidneys under reduced oxygen supply in the body (e.g. at an altitude of about or above 2,000 m, where the air is rarified). Via the bloodstream, erythropoietin reaches the bone-marrow cells and activates them to produce more red blood cells (erythrocytes). This increases the amount of the oxygen-transporting protein (hemoglobin) and, consequently, improves the oxygen supply to tissues. Some believe this normal mechanism of adaptation may be used to increase the aerobic capacity and, thereby, the chances to win a competition. Erythropoietin is not easily available and, therefore, some athletes use *blood doping* instead. Blood doping means transfusion or reinfusion of blood 1 or 2 days before a competition [22]. The first documented transfusion for such purpose was that in American cyclists during the 1976 Montreal Olympic Games [1]. So far there is no commonly shared proof of increased performance due to erythropoietin or blood doping [22, 23]. The health risks were documented, though: 3 of the 7 American cyclists with blood transfusion fell ill. Health risks include fever, hepatitis or AIDS infection, circulation overload and even death if incompatible blood is transfused. For these reasons erythropoietin injection and blood transfusion are forbidden in sports.

Adrenocorticotropic hormone (corticotropin, ACTH; available as Acethropan, Actargel, Cortrosyn, Synacthen, etc.) is a hormone of the anterior pituitary gland. It reaches the adrenal cortex through the bloodstream and stimulates the production of specific type of steroid hormones, called *corticosteroids*. The effect of ACTH injection is, therefore, similar to that of corticosteroid hormones. Normally, these hormones are vital. Their medical use is determined by their potent anti-inflammatory, anti-allergic and antishock effects. Besides, they produce euphoria and glycogen accumulation in the liver and muscles. This is an attractive reason for their use in sports. The resulting glycogen accumulation is, unfortunately, due to protein degradation.

The other effects are even more undesirable. They include steroid diabetes, bleeding ulcers in the stomach and intestines, bone demineralization with ensuing fractures and even epileptiform convulsions. For these reasons ACTH injection is forbidden, as is the oral or parenteral administration of corticosteroids. In some cases, however, athletes may have medical indications for corticosteroid treatment. These include treatment of inflammatory and allergic diseases of the eyes and ears (drops and ointments for external use), skin diseases, inhalations for asthma and allergic rhinitis and intra-articular injections for diseases of the joints. In all such cases an authorized person (the team doctor) must submit a written report to the IOC Medical Commission stating the diagnosis, the drug and doses used, and the mode of application. If he fails to do so, the anti-doping regulations will be enforced.

Doping Control Procedures: Right and Responsibilities of Athletes

Sample Collection

The first four athletes by placing in the final contest are tested. Moreover, additional competitors may also be checked at random. They shall be selected by drawing lots. An athlete may be tested for doping on more than one occasion during the different stages of the competition.

The competitor selected for a doping check shall be handed a special testing notification by a representative of the Organizing Committee. From that moment on he shall be attended by the representative of the Organizing Committee to the waiting room of the station where the sample shall be taken. The competitor has the right to request the presence of an attendant from his delegation (coach, doctor, team official or his representative). The doping control notification shall have the competitor's starting number filled in, and the place and hour of reporting. The notification must have a detachable stub with the competitor's starting number also written on it. The competitor shall show his identity card and confirm by his signature on the stub that he is notified of the place and time of reporting. If he fails to report then the case shall be submitted to the IOC Medical Commission. The competitor must also be warned of the possible consequences should he fail or refuse to report for control.

Upon arrival at the doping control station the competitor and the accompanying persons (representative of the Organizing Committee and a representative of the competitor's team) shall hand the stub to the official responsible for doping control, and shall be attended by a member of the doping control team. The competitor's name and starting number (certified by his personal identity card), the time of arrival and other necessary notes shall be entered in the records.

Only one competitor at a time shall be called into the office for doping control. The accompanying person, the official in charge of the doping station, a representative of the international federation concerned, a member of the IOC Medical Commission, the medical technician keeping the records, the official in charge of taking samples and an interpreter if required, have the right to be present in the doping control office.

The competitor shall select a plastic container with two wide-neck glass bottles. They shall bear identical code numbers with A and B etched on each one, respectively. The competitor shall take them personally to the sample-collection room. He/she shall urinate into bottle A (at least 75 ml) under the supervision of the responsible person. The competitor shall then go back to the office, carrying bottle A containing the urine sample and the plastic container with bottle B. Under the supervision of the competitor the medical technician shall transfer 1/3 of the urine sample into bottle B and shall close both bottles securely. The competitor has the right to perform this manipulation should he/she wish to do so.

The competitor shall select one bag A (blue) and one bag B (yellow) into which the urine bottles shall be placed. He/she shall also select a pair of plastic coded seals. The technician shall place the card bearing the seal code and the code etched on the bottle in the respective window of blue bag A and yellow bag B. The bottles are closed securely and placed in the respective bag and sealed with the appropriate coded seal (blue seal and blue bag for bottle A, yellow seal and yellow bag for bottle B). The competitor and the accompanying person have the right to make sure that the bags are correctly sealed, the control cards are correct, and the numbers in the records correspond to those on the cards. Then the competitor shall sign the records certifying that the whole procedure is correct, or he may enter his objections. The records shall also be signed by the official in charge of doping control, by the accompanying person, and by the representatives of the IOC Medical Commission and international federation if they are present. Every single copy of the records shall be placed into a separate envelope bearing the code numbers of the seals of bag A (blue) and bag B (yellow). The envelope is closed and sealed in the presence of the accompanying person, and the officials mentioned above shall place their signatures on it. An envelope shall be opened only under permission by the official representative of the President of the IOC Medical Commission.

Finally, the technician in charge of the doping control procedure shall place all sealed bags A (blue) in a blue transport container and all sealed bags B (yellow) in a yellow transport container. The containers shall be sealed with the numbered seal of the respective color in the presence of a representative of the IOC Medical Commission. A special courier shall take the sealed containers to the laboratory where the samples shall be analyzed.

Sample Analysis

The samples shall be analyzed according to the methods and techniques adopted by the IOC Medical Commission. The analysis may be performed only in one of the IOC accredited laboratories, where its quality is in conformity with the highest world standards. These laboratories are subject to testing several times a year in order to guarantee the quality and reliability of their work.

Should the analysis of sample A establish the presence of a banned substance, an official representative of the IOC Medical Commission shall inform by letter the head of the competitor's team. This letter shall also indicate the date and hour of the control analysis, i.e. the analysis of the urine sample in bottle B.

The analysis of sample B shall be performed in the same laboratory by another team and under the supervision of the IOC Medical Commission representative. The competitor's delegation has the right to send three representatives to attend the analysis of sample B. The analysis of sample B shall be considered final. Should it confirm the positive result the representative of the IOC Medical Commission shall call a meeting at which the competitor is invited to give his/her explanations on the case. The final decision of the sanctions shall be made by the IOC Executive Committee.

All this detail exists to be absolutely certain the competitors rights are fully protected. Accredited laboratories can identify banned drugs even when they are present in amounts less than one millionth of a gram. In addition, the sample-taking procedure is supervised during all its stages by the competitor himself. The competitors interests are also protected by the fact because experienced and knowledgeable representatives can attend the entire analysis, including the control analysis of sample B. Finally, decisions on sanctions are discussed at national and international level by highly qualified experts.

Tentative List of the Most Commonly Used Banned Drugs

This list is based on a fundamental publication and shows the systemic name of the active substance and the names of the pharmaceutical preparations containing it, given in parentheses [3].

Stimulants

(1) Amfepramone (Adiposan, Anorex, Brendalit, Dietec, Dietil, Frekentine, Lineal-Rivo, Linea-Valeas, Lipomin, Liposlim, Magrene, Magrex Retard, Menutil, Moderatan, Nulobes, Prefamone, Regenon, Regibon, Slim-Plus, Tenucap, Tepanil).

(2) Amphetamine (Aktedrin, Aktedron, Amphedrine, Benzedrine, Benzpramine, Centramina, Euphodyn, Leptamine, Monophos, Phenedrine Profetamine, Psychoton, Raphetamine, Ro-Diet, Simpamine, Simpatina).

(3) Bemegride (Ahypnon, Antibarb, Etimid, Glutamisol, Malysol, Megibal, Medimid, Nikedimide).

(4) Caffeine (Aceffein, Aflukin-Grippe Tabletten, Anapyrin, Antibex, Antigripal, Antigrippalin, Asthma-frenon S, Avamigran N, Benalgin, Cafaspin, Cafergot N, Callergin, Celetil, Chephapyrin N, Cinalgin, Cofaminol, Coffalon, Coffetylin, Corvipas, Ditonal, Dolviran, Entrodyn, Ergo-Lonasid, Euvitan, Fineural N, Gentarol N, Gentil, Gewodyn, Grippostad C, Herbin-Stodin Schmerztabletten, Ilvico N, Kola-Dallmann, Kontragripp, Kreuz-Tabletten, Lonarid N, Mandros, Mega-Dolor, Mi-

graenex, Miophen, Neo-Gepan, Optalidon, Paracofdal, Percofledrinol N, Pharmazon, Praecimol, Prontopyrin, Kopfschmerzen Refagan N, Riperol, Romigal N, Saridon, Sedalgin, Sedaphen, Siguran N retard, Theophedrin, Thomapyrin, Veralgit).

(5) Cathine (Adiposetten, Amorphan, Boxogetten, Exponcit, Gracil, Lorenz Schoenschlank, Miniscap, Minusin, Mirapront N, Myocoryl, Neo-Soldana, Norapress, Plevent, Raucherstop, Recatol, Reduform, Schlank-Dragees).

(6) Ephedrine (Alfabet Schlankheitsdragees, Afra-Hustentropfen, Antussan, Apracur, Asthma 'Berco', Asthma-Bisolvon, Asthma-Frenon, Asthmin, Asthmodem, Asthmolysin, Cephedrin, Codyl, Coldorgan, Dicton, Dorex, Efisalin, Elero, Endrine, Endemol, Ephetonin, Equsil, Fagusal, Fomagrippin, Grippocaps, Hustagil, Hypotonin, Ipalat, Keldrin, Kuronde, Lidocaton, Liquemin Depot, Makatussin forte, Mandrogripp, Miktiplon, Mintusin, Mirfusot, Morasthman, Mucron, Nasalgon, Neocor, Neo-Felsol, Neuridal, Noordyl, Normotin, Noxenur, Optipect, Pectamed, Perdiphen, Perspiran, Pertussin, Pharhin, Piniol, Praecipect, Priatan, Pro-Pecton, Pulmocordio, Respirogutt, Rhinamid, Rhinosine, Rhino-Xylidrin, Scopedal, Sirthyco, Solamin, Solgen, Tecoryl, Thymipin, Thymitussin, Tiffanova, Tolusot, Tonaton, Tussamag, Tussipect, Vitenur).

(7) Etilefrine (Amphodyn, Dihydergot, Effortil, Ergolefrin, Ethylfron, Fetano, Hyurina, Influbene, Presoton, Pulsamin, Thomasin).

(8) Ethamivan (Cactus, Card-Instenon, Clairvan, Corvanil, Emivan, Instenon, Romecor, Tonolift Efeka, Vallamida, Vandid).

(9) Heptaminol (Altocor, Amidrina, Ampecyclal, Arcor, Bascardial, Bayrotren, Bronchovis, Cortensor, Eoden, Eptavigor, Funesil, Heptylon, Myolytril, Ortho-heptamin, Paretocard, Veno-Hexanicit, Veno-Tebonin).

(10) Methylphenidate (Centedrine, Metylofenidan, Ritaline).

(11) Nikethamide (Anacardone, Analeptin, Cardiamin, Coramin, Corazon, Cordalept, Corditon, Coral, Corvital, Cormed, Eucoran, Glucardiamid, Hypotonin, Juvacor, Kardonyl, Miocardina, Neo-Felsol, Nicamide, Nicorine, Percoral, Tonocard, Tonus, Vasazol, Vitamin-Schlanktropfen, Zellaforte).

(12) Pentetrazol (Afpred, Angiasol, Cardiazol, Centrazole, Corazol, Corasid, Corvasol, Deumacard, Leptazol, Metrazol, Pentrazol, Veriazol).

(13) Phentermine (Adipex, Adipo II, Aneroxina, Dapex, Duromina, Fastin, Ionokraft, Ionamin, Levum, Linyl, Lipopill, Minicaps, Minobese, Mirapront, Netto-Longcaps, Oby-Trim, Ona-Mas, Panbesy Nyscaps, Parmine, Phentermyl Wyncaps, Phentrol, Phermin, Reducyl, Rolaphent, Tor, Umi-Pex, Wilpo, Wilpor-Clear).

(14) Phenylephrine (Adrianol, Alcon-Efril, Allerest, Almefrin, Biomeydrin, Caltheon, Degest, Dristan, Fenilfar, Fenox, Glanco-Biciron,

Isophrine, Isopto, Melbit, Metaoxedrin, Mobilat Sportgel, Moroven, Mud-
frin, Naldecol, Nasophen, Neo Synephrine, Neophryn, Noflu F, Nostril,
Ozabran, Pyracort D, Rhinex, Rhinivit, Rhinocaps, Rinisol, Snup, Synasal,
Trimedil, Tussidan, Tylex, Vistaprefrin, Vistosan).

(15) Pholedrine (Adyston, Kontragripp, Pentavenon, Pressistan, Pul-
sotyl, Venosan, Veriazol, Veritol, Zellaforte).

(16) Prenylamine (Agosol, Angiovigor, Angorsan, Bismetin, Car-
dional, Corontin, Corosten, Crepasin, Daxauten, Epocol, Ercapsil, Euca-
dion, Falicor, Herzcon, Hoechst 12512, Hostaginan, Incoran, Irrorin,
Lactamine, Newsantine, Nyuple, Onlemin, Plactamin, Rausetin, Reocoryn,
Roinin, Sedolatan, Segontin, Synadrin, Vasangor).

(17) Pseudoephedrine (Afrinol, Besan, First Sing, Galpseud, Halofed,
Linctifed, Neo-Synephrinol, Novafed, Oranyl, Otrinol, Profedrine, Ro-
bidrine, Sinufed, Sudafed, Sudrin).

(18) Strychnine (Calmicor, Cardioregis, Circyvit, Dysurgal, Morillen,
Moro-Herzwein, Silberpillen, Spasmofuga, Sulfa-Dysurgal, Tonol, Vertc-
bran N).

Note: The use of caffeine-containing tablets is not absolutely forbidden. Do not take more than one tablet as a single dose, however, otherwise
the caffeine concentration in urine will exceed the permissible limit. Always
check for other banned drugs in a caffeine-containing preparation!

Narcotics
(1) Codeine (Benadryl, Bisolvomed m.C., Bisolvon-Gribletten,
Bromapect forte, Bronchoforton c.C., Compretten, Codicaps, Codicept,
Codicompren retard, Codidoxal, Codipertussin, Codipront, Codterpin,
Contrancural N, Dolviran, Ephcodral, Ergo-Lonarid, Euspasmin, Gentarol
N, Hypertussin S/K, Lonarid N, Mandros forte, Medocodene, Mega-Dolor,
Migraeflux N, Migraene-Kranit, Miophen, Nedelon, Neurodyne, Panadeine
Co, Paracodal, Paracofdal, Paradeine, Paralgin, Pardale, Pectinfant N,
Praecimed N, Precineural, Propain, Sedalgin, Solpadein, Spasmo-Cibalgin
comp.S, Spasmo-Gentarol N, Syndol, Toximer, Veganin, Veralgit).

(2) Dextropropoxyphene (Abalgin, Cosalgesic, Depronal SA, Dolene
Plaine, Dolocap, Doloksen, Dolorphen, Dolotard, Doloxene, Dolo-Neu-
trat, Dolo-Prolixan, Doraphen HCL, Mardon, Margesic Improved, Pro-
pox, Propoxychel, Proxagesic, Proxene, Rosimon-neu, Scrip-Dyne, Develin
retard, Dextrogesic, Distalgesic, Dolo-Neurotrat, Doloxen, Ultrapyrin).

(3) Dihydrocodeine (Antibex, Codhydrine, DHC Continus, Makatussin, Monacant, Monapax, Paracodin, Tiamon).

(4) Dipipanone (Diconal, Pipadone, Wellconal).

(5) Ethylmorphine (Beldipin, Codethyline, Cosylan, Diolan, Dionin,
Diosan, Dipidolor, Neo-Codion, Pulmorex, Tussedat, Tussirol).

(6) Hydrocodone (Biocodone, Codinova, Corutol, Didrale, Dihydrocodeinon Streuli, Hycodan, Hycon, Hydrocon, Novicodina, Synconin).

(7) Methadone (Adolan, Althose, Amidon, Cloro Nona, Deprodol, Disket, Doloheptan, Dolophine, Eptadone, Heptadon, Heptanal, Heptanon, Ketalgin, Mephenon, Metasedin, Methadose, Physeptone, Polamidon, Sedamidone, Sedo Rapide, Symoron, Tussol, Westadone).

(8) Morphine (Contalgen, Dosette, Duramorph PF, Duromorph, MS Contin, MST Mundipharma, Mundidol, Nepenthe, Nubain, Omnopone, Pantopon, Roxanol, Theba-Intran).

(9) Oxycodone (Boncodal, Dinarcon, Eudone, Eudol, Eucodal, Oxanest, Proladone, Roxicodone, Supendol).

(10) Pethidine (Algil, Alodan, Centralgin, Dolanquifa, Dolantin, Dolargan, Dolestine, Dolisina, Doloneurin, Dolosal, Dolsin, Dosette Meperidine, Mefedina, Pethadol, Pethidol, Pethoid, Pro-Meperdan, Psyquil comp., Suppolosal, Tubex Meperidine).

Anabolic-Androgenic Steroids

(1) Boldenone (Boldan Equipoise, Parenabol, Vebonol).

(2) Clostebol (Alfa-Trofedermin, Megagrisevit, Steranabol, Test-Anabol.

(3) Fluoxymesterone (Afluteston, Androsterolo, Halotestin, Ora-Testryl U-gono, Ultandren).

(4) Mesterolone (Androviron, Mestoran, Pluriviron, Proviron, Vistimon).

(5) Methandienone (Andoredan, Crein, Dianabol, Metanabol, Naposim, Nevrobolettae, Nerobol, Perabol, Vanabol).

(6) Methenolone (Primobolan, Primobolan S).

(7) Methyltestosterone (Android, Androteston, Bonaclimax, Gynosteron, Methandren, Testred, Testovis, Zimba forte).

(8) Nandrolone (Adenocorin, Anaboline, Anabosan, Anticatabolin, Anadur, Decabolin, Deca-Duraboline, Deca-Noralone, Decolone, Durabol, Durabolin, Dynabolon, Fortabolin, Hybolin, Methybol-Depot, Nerobolil, Norstenol, Palactin, Retabolil, Sanabolicum, Sintabolin, Sterobolin, Strabolene, Turinabol, Ziremilon).

(9) Oxandrolone (Anavar, Antitriol, Lonavar, Vasorome).

(10) Oxymetholone (Anadrol, Anapolon, Anasteron, Android, Dynasten, Hemogenin, Nastenon, Plenastril, Synasteron, Zenalosyn).

(11) Stanozolol (Anasyth, Anazole, Stromba, Strombaject, Tevabolin, Winsteroid, Winstrol).

(12) Testosterone (Agovirin, Andriol, Androfort, Androlin, Androtardyl, Anertan, Arderon, Delatest, Durandron, Enarmon, Femovirin, Homosteron, Hydrotest, Lyandron, Malogen, Malogex, Omnadren, Primo-

dian Depot, Primoteston Depot, Reposteron, Retandrol, Sustanon, Triolandren, Testes-Uvocal, Testoviron, Undestor, Virormone).

Beta-Blockers

(1) Acebutolol (Acecor, Acetanol, Alol, Diasectral, Nolson, Neptal, Prent 400, Sectral, Tredalat, Wesrfalin).

(2) Alprenolol (Antra, Apllobal, Aptin, Aptol, Betacard, Elperl, Gubernal, Regletin).

(3) Atenolol (Blokium, Ibinolo, Myocord, Nif-Ten, Normiten, Ormidol, Prenormin, Prinorm, Seles Beta, Tri-Normin, Vericordin).

(4) Labetalol (Abetol, Alfabetal, Amipress, Ipolab, Labelol, Labitex, Labrocol, Liondox, Lolum, Normodyne, Presdate, Presolol, Salmagne, Tenormin).

(5) Metoprolol (Beprolo, Betabloc, Bloksan, Inophyllin, Lopresor, Neobloc, Prelis, Seloken).

(6) Oxprenolol (Captol, Cordexol, Coretal, Dialicor, Evinrozit, Flecor, Oxanol, Ranidrex, Rixiprol, Secondafil, Trasicor, Vrachor, Zetonium).

(7) Pindolol (Barbloc, Redrenal, Betapindol, Calvisken, Cocaserln, Decreten, Durapindol, Nitrisken, Pectobloc, Pinbetol, Pindomex, Pinbloc, Treparasen, Viskaldix, Viskene, Visken-Quinze).

(8) Propranolol (Avlocardyl, Bedranol, Berkolol, Betaprol, Betares, Betaryl, Beta-Neg, Beta-Tablinen, Beta-Timelets, Cardinaol, Ciplar, Deralin, Detensol, Dideral, Dociton, Efectolol, Elbrol, Euchon, Frekven, Frina, Inderal, Indobloc, Kodtalerg, Nedis, Neopranol, Noloten, Novopranol, Obsidan, Palisan, Panolol, Pebarol Pranix, Pranolol, Prano-Puren, Prolol, Pronovan, Propabloc, Propalong, Propranur, Pur-Blocka, Pylapron, Reducor, Sagittol, Sawatal, Sloprolol, Wancoton, Ziserfin).

(9) Sotalol (Betades, Beta-Cardone, Jusotal, Lesotal, Sotacor, Sotalex, Sotapor).

(10) Timolol (Betim, Blocadren, Calvisken, Cardina, Carvisken, Chibro-Timoptol, Cusimolol, Imolate, Normabel, Noval-Ofal, Proflax, Temserin, Timacar, Timacor, Timoptol, Yesan).

Diuretics

(1) Acetazolamide (Acetamid, Acetamox, Acetazolam, Ailopan, Albox, Atenezol, Cetazol, Defiltran, Diamox, Edemox, Epilemide, Glauconox, Glaupax, Hydrazol, Ledriamox, Natrionex, Nephramid, Oedemin, Renamid, Uramox, Zolmax).

(2) Amiloride (Amiclaran, Amiduret, Amilco Burg, Amiloretic, Aquaretic Arumil, Bercamil, Colectril, Diursan, Durarese, Esmalorid, Hy-

drocomp-Tablinen, Kaluril, Midamor, Modamide, Moducrin, Moduretic, Nirulid, Pandiuren, Puritrid, Refluin, Tensoflux).

(3) Bendroflumethiazide (Aprinox, Benuron, Benzide, Berkozide, Bristuric, Centyl, Esberizide, Flumesil, Idrexan-NA, Naturetin, Naturine-Leo, Neo Naclex, Notens, Pluryle, Poliuron, Sali-Aldopur Salural, Salures, Seda-Ripicin, Tensoflux, Urizid).

(4) Bumetanide (Aneiromox, Aquazonz, Diurama, Lixil-Leo, Lune-toron, Salurex, Salurin, Segurex).

(5) Chlormerodrine (Asahydrin, Bucohydral, Diuros, Mercloran, Mercoral, Merculest, Merilid, Neohydrin, Novohydrin, Oricur, Orimercur, Ormerdan).

(6) Chlortalidone (Aquadon, Dareb-n, Higroton, Hydopan, Hydro-long, Hypertol, Igrolina, Igroton, Impresso-Puren, Novothalidone, Oede-mase-long, Prelis comp., Renon, Servidone, Thalitone, Urandil, Urid, Uridon).

(7) Ethacrynic acid (Crinuryl, Edecril, Edecrin, Hydromedin, Tola-dren, Uregyt).

(8) Furosemide (Accent, Aisemide, Aluzine, Arasemide, Betasemid, Diaterene F, Desal, Desdemin, Diaphal, Dimazon, Disal, Discord, Diural, Diuresal, Diurix, Diurasa, Diusemide, Diutensat, Diutrix, Dryptal, Dura-furid, Duraspiron, Edemid, Egotux, Errolon, Furosemin, Frusetic, Frusid, Fuluvamide, Furanthral, Furanthril, Furesis, Furetic, Furex, Furix, Furomex, Furorese, Furose, Furesedon, Furoside, Fusid, Geimonil, Hy-drotrix, Hydro-rapid Tablinen, Impugan, Inzury, Ipodiuril, Kaltex, Ked-itrol, Kutrix, Ladonna, Lasiletten, Lasilix, Lasix, Laxur, Lizik, Lowpston, Macasirool, Menol, Neosemide, Neo-Renal, Nephron, Nicoral, Nortensin, Novosemide, Oedemase, Oedemex, Panseman, Polysquall A, Promedes, Protargen, Puresis, Radiamin, Radonna, Rasisemid, Retep, Rosemide, Seguril, Semid, Sigasalur, Tabilon-A, Terbolan, Tex, Transit, Trofurit, Uremide, Urenil, Urex, Uritol).

(9) Hydrochlorothiazide (Adelphan-Esidrex, Amiduret, Amilo Burg, Amiloretic, Amilo-Recip comp., Aquaretic, Betathiazid, Beta-Nephral, Calmoserpin, Catiazada, Chemhydrazide, Chlorzide, Chlothia, Cloredema, Deidran, Delco Retic, Diaqua, Dichlorosal, Dichlotride, Didral, Dihydran, Direma, Disalunil, Dithiazid, Diu 25 Voigt, Diu Tonolytril, Diu Veno-stasin, Diuchlor H, Diureticum Verla, Diurogen, Diursana H, Diu-melusin, Dixidrasi, Di-Chlotride, Duradiuret, Elfanex, Esidrex, Esidrix, Esimil, Es-iteren, Esoidrina, Exidrin, Fluvin, Hydrosaluretil, Hyclozid, Hydoril, Hy-drazide, Hydrex, Hydrite, Hydrodiuretex, Hydrodiuril, Hydromal, Hydro-saluret, Hydrosaluric, Hydro-Diuril, Hyperetic, Hypothiazid, Hytrid, Idrodi-uvis, Idrofluin, Ivangan, Kenazide, Lexor, Loqua, Manimon, Manuril, Maschitt, Moduretic, Moilarorin, Natrimax, Nefrol, Neo-Cloruril, Neo-

Codema, Neo-Flumen, Neo-Saluretic, Nephral, Neutolide, Novodiurex, Novohydrazide, Olivysat, Olmagran, Oretic, Pantemon, Panurin, Raucombin, Regulaserp, Ranifluss, Resaltex, Rhefluin, Risicordin, Rozide, Salcant, Saldiuril, Sali-Puren, Slimin, Tenzide, Thiadril, Thiaretic, Thiuretic, Urirex).

(10) Spironolactone (Acelat, Airolactone, Aldace, Aldactone, Aldonar, Aldopur, Aldospirone, Altex, Aporason, Aquareduct, Deveron, Diatensec, Diakton, Dira, Elmion, Hokulaton, Idrolatt Euteberol, Idrolattone, Localmin, Lacdene, Laractone, Nefurofan, Osiren, Osyrol, Penantin, Plarenyl, Practon, Risicordin, Rolactone, Sagisal, Sali-Aldopur, Servilactone, Sincomen, Spironal, Spiresis, Spiretic, Spiridon, Spirix, Spiro, Spiroctan, Spirodigal, Spirolang, Spirolone, Spiron, Spironothiazid, Spiropal, Spirostada, Spirotone, Sprionolacton, Supra-Puren, Suracton, Uractone, Uridactone).

(11) Triamterene (Atensolan, Betathiazid, Beta-Nephral, Beta-Turfa, Calmoserpin, Dehydrosanol, Diesse, Diu Tonolytril, Diu Venostasin, Diucomp, Diurene, Diureticum Verba, Diutensat, Diutrix, Duradiuret, Duraspiron, Dyrenium, Dytac, Dytide H, Esiteren, Furesis comp., Hydrotrix, Jatropur, Kalistat, Manimon, Natrium, Neotri, Nephral, Renifluss, Resaltex, Salcant, Sali-Puren, Slimin, Teriam, Triarene, Triazid, Urethren, Urocaudal).

Tentative List of Allowed Drugs and Drug Preparations

Antacids and Drugs Against Diarrhea and Peptic Ulcers
Acinorm, Alcap, Aldrox, Allulose, Altacit, Aludrox, Aluminox, Amphojel, Andursil, Antepsin, Biogastron, Burimamide, Cantil, Cimetum, Colofac, Diarsed, Diloran, Diovol, Donnagel, Duspatal, Equilet, Gamma-gel, Gastridine, Gastromet, Gaviscon, Gelusil, Imodium, Kaomycin, Kaopectate, Lomotil, Maalox, Metiamide, Metoclol, Milid, Palmicol, Pepto-Bismol, Primperan, Prodexin, Promid, Reasec, Reglan, Rinveral, Riopan, Riopone, Robalate, Sulcrate, Tagamet, Talcid, Titralac, Ulcerban, Ulcermin, Ulsanic, Unigest, Zantac.

Drugs Against Nausea and Vomiting
Anaus, Antivert, Aviomarine, Bonamine, Dramamine, Emetrol, Gravol, Ibikin, Neptusan, Nibromin-A, Postafen, Stemetil, Tigan, Torecan, Vertigon, Vomex A, Yesdol, Yophadol.

Anti-Asthmatic and Anti-Allergic Agents
(1) Allowed as aerosol formulations for inhalation: Albuterol, Alotec, Alupent, Asmaten, Asmatol, Asmidon, Astmopent, Astop, Beconase, Becotide, Bitoltcrol, Bricalin, Bricanyl, Bristurin, Dosalupent, Fecvone, Metaprel, Pulmadil, Salbutan, Salbutol, Sultanol, Terbasmin, Ventolin.

(2) Allowed regardless of the formulation: Aldecin, Aminodur, Asmafil, Atrovent, Beclovent, Bronkodyl, Cardophyllin, Choledyl, Corophyllin, Euphyllin, Euspirax, Theocoline, Theo-Dur, Theolair, Theovent.

(3) Other antihistamine preparations: Actidil, Actidilon, Allergex, Alusas, Anthisan, Antistin, Astemizole, Atalis-D, Atarax, Atosil, Avomine, Azaron, Banistyl, Bonpac, C-Meton-S, Chlorpheniramine, Chlor-Tripolon, Clistin, Dimetane, Di-paralene, Ebolin, Fabhistin, Histamanal, Histalert, Histanil, Histex, Histaryl, Homadamon, Idulamine, Ifrasarl, Incidal, Lecasol, Lenazine, Migristene, Nuran, Omeril, Optimine, Periactin, Peritol, Phenergan, Polaronil, Promaquid, Pyribenzamine, Pyrimetane, Reconin, Sacronal, Seldane, Tavegyl, Tavist, Teldane, Trihistan, Triludan, Trimeton, Venen.

Drugs Used to Treat Coughs
(1) Syrup formulations: Balminil DM, Bisolvon, Cosylan, Dextphan, Reorganin, Resyl, Robitussin plain, Sancos.
(2) Tablets: Astomin, Balminil, Bisolvon, Bractos, Bradosal, Cepacol, Coricidin throat lozenges, Hustazol, Lysobex, Merocets, Neo-Bradoral, Respirex, Sinecod, Tessalin, Tessalon.

Decongestants and Nasal Preparations
Afrazine, Beconase, Iliadin, Lidil, Nafrine, Naphazoline, Nasivin, Otrivin, Rynacrom, Soframycin, Tyzine.

Non-Narcotic Analgesics and Non-Steroidal Anti-Inflammatory Agents
Acetamol, Acetard, Acetylin, Adiro, Alcacyl, Allopydin, Aluprin, Anaprox, Aquaprin, Arlef, Asatard, Aspasol, Aspirin, Benortan, Benotabol, Ben-U-Ron, Bonabol, Brufen, Bufemid, Calip, Capisten, Cinnamin, Cinopal, Clinoril, Cresopirine, Desinflam, Dirox, Dispril, Dolisal, Dolobid, Dorbid, Ecotrin, Ennagesis, Enteretas, Entrophen, Enzamin, Feldene, Flanax, Flosint, Glifanan, Hyprin, Idarac, Imotryl, Indacin, Indocid, Istopirine, Motrin, Naixan, Nalfon, Naprosyn, Norfemac, Orudis, Paloxin, Panadol, Paramidin, Pasolin, Pentosol, Ponstan, Ponstel, Pontal, Prinalgin, Profenid, Progesic, Prolix, Prolixan, Rheumox, Rhonal, Salitison, Sedapyren, Sulindac, Superpyrin, Tamas, Tandearil, Tanderil, Tantum, Tolectin, Tylenol, Voltaren, Winolate, Zubirol, Zumaril.

Sedatives and Tranquillizers
Abasin, Adalin, Amytal, Ativan, Brovarin, Chloralol, Dalmadorm, Dalmane, Dalmate, Doriden, Dormogen, Equanil, Euhypnos, Evidorm, Evipan, Gardenal, Halcion, Haldol, Largactil, Levanxol, Lexotanil, Librium, Mebaral, Medomin, Mogadon, Nembutal, Noludar, Noctec,

Normison, Prominal, Restoril, Restwel, Schlafen, Serenid, Serepax, Sobile, Soneryl, Sopental, Stelazine, Tranxene, Tuinal, Valium, Volamin.

Contraceptives
Anacyclin, Brevinor, Conova 30, Demulen 50, Eugynon, Exlutona, Femulen, Micronovum, Minilyn, Nordiol, Ortho-novum, Ovostat, Ovral, Ovulen.

References

1 Dubin CL: Report of the Commission of Inquiry into the Use of Drugs and Banned Practices Intended to Increase Athletic Performance. Ottawa, Canadian Government Publishing Centre, 1990.
2 Porrit A: Doping. J Sports Med Phys Fitness 1965;5:166.
3 Donike M, Rauth S: Dopingkontrollen. Köln, Bundesinstitut für Sportwissenschaft, 1990.
4 Powers SK, Dodd S: Caffeine and endurance performance. Sports Med 1985;2:165–174.
5 Kochakian CD, Murlin JR: The effect of male hormones on the protein and energy metabolism of castrate dogs. J Nutr 1935;10:437–458.
6 Wade N: Anabolic steroids: Doctors denounce them, but athletes aren't listening. Science 1972;176:1399–1403.
7 American College of Sports Medicine: Position stand on the use of anabolic-androgenic steroids in sports. Med Sci Sports Exerc 1987;19:534–538.
8 Wright JE: Anabolic steroids and athletes. Exerc Sport Sci Rev 1980;8:149–202.
9 Kilshaw BH, Harkness RA, Hobson BM, Smith AWM: The effects of large doses of the anabolic steroid, methandrostenolone, on an athlete. Clin Endocrinol 1975;4:537–541.
10 Keul J, Deus H, Kinderman W: Anabole hormone: Schädigung, Leistungsfähigkeit und Stoffwechsel. Med Klin 1976;71:497–503.
11 Yesalis CE III, Wright JE, Bahrke MS: Epidemiological and policy issues in the measurement of the long-term health effects of anabolic-androgenic steroids. Sports Med 1989;8:129–138.
12 Ishak K: Hepatic neoplasms associated with contraceptive and anabolic steroids. Rec Res Cancer Res 1979;66:73–128.
13 Shapiro P, Ikedo RM, Ruebner BH, Conners MH, Halsted CC, Abildgaan CF: Multiple hepatic tumors and peliosis hepatis in Fanconi's anemia treated with androgens. Am J Dis Child 1977;131:1104–1106.
14 Martikainen H, Alen M, Rahkila P, Vihko R: Testicular responsiveness to human chorionic gonadotropin during transient hypogonadotropic hypogonadism induced by androgenic anabolic steroids in power athletes. J Steroid Biochem 1986;25:109–112.
15 Schurmeyer T, Knuth UA, Berkien L, Nieschlag E: Reversible azoospermia induced by the anabolic steroid 19-nortestosterone. Lancet 1984;i:417–420.
16 Alen M, Rahkila P: Anabolic-androgenic steroid effects on endocrinology and lipid metabolism in athletes. Sports Med 1988;6:327–332.
17 Reeves RD, Morris MD, Barbour GI: Hyperlipidemia due to oxymetholone therapy. JAMA 1976;236:464–472.
18 Webb OL, Laskarzewski PM, Glueck CJ: Severe depression of high-density lipoprotein cholesterol levels in weightlifters and body builders by self-administered exogeneous testosterone and anabolic-androgenic steroids. Metabolism 1984;33:971–975.

19   McNutt R: Acute myocardial infarction in a 22-years old world class weightlifter using anabolic steroids. Am J Cardiol 1988;62:164.
20   MacIntyre JG: Growth hormone and athletes. Sports Med 1987;4:129–140.
21   Goldberg AL, Goodman HM: relationship between growth hormone and muscle work in determining muscle size. J Physiol 1969;200:655–666.
22   American College of Sports Medicine: Position stand on blood doping as an ergogenic aid. Med Sci Sports Exerc 1987;19:540–543.
23   Spriet LL, Gledhill N, Froese AB, Wilkes DL: Effect of graded erythrocytemia on cardiovascular and metabolic responses to exercise. J Appl Physiol 1986;61:1942–1948.

Prof. Emmanuel P. Gachev, MD, DSc Department of Biochemistry,
National Academy of Sports, Doping Control Laboratory,
Research Centre of Sports, Sofia 1172 (Bulgaria)

Karvonen J, Lemon PWR, Iliev I (eds): Medicine in Sports Training and Coaching.
Med Sport Sci. Basel, Karger, 1992, vol 35, pp 49–68

Environmental Adaptation and Physical Training

Juha Karvonen

Department of Clinical Physiology, University Hospital of Tampere, Finland

Contents

Introduction

When one travels far abroad, new environmental, temperature and weather conditions, together with a delay in adapting to a different time zone, decrease performance capacity initially. Through adaptation, this original capacity is gradually restored. People normally living in a cool climate perform less well in heavy exercise when the weather is suddenly warm. In principle, performance capacity also decreases when one moves rapidly from hot to a cold or cool climate.

In a hot climate before acclimatization one produces smaller volumes of sweat with relatively high salt contents. With acclimatization sweat rate is increased and the electrolyte concentration is decreased. Core temperature and heart rate are higher during exertion before acclimatization as a sign of heat stress.

Some of the mechanisms regulating adaptation to cold and to heat are similar. Cold weather causes fluid and electrolyte (salt) loss due to increased urinary output. This leads to a diminished blood volume, which taxes the heart and reduces performance capacity. Many people living in a cold climate, such as the Lapps, take salt instead of sugar in their coffee: this probably helps in maintaining the fluid-electrolyte balance in the cold climate.

Travelling to another continent often means changing time zones and, therefore, disturbing the hormonal circadian rhythms. Crossing a few time zones will probably not reduce performance capacity. Primarily, jet lag occurs when crossing four or more time zones. Travelling occurs too rapidly for bodily rhythms to adapt to the new time. This is a common phenomenon in the present era of flying. However, the decrease in performance capacity due to jet lag does not continue as long as with heat or cold stress.

The Heat Regulation System

The human body has a heat regulation system that during rest keeps the core temperature between 36.0 and 37.3 °C in ambient temperatures of 10–55 °C when air humidity and wind velocity are favorable. Increased humidity and wind speed notably restrict the range of tolerable ambient temperatures [1].

Skin temperature is lower than deep body temperature, and it decreases from the trunk towards the extremities. In cold environments finger temperature may be ten degrees below that at the shoulder. Thermoregulation is related to the dynamic balance between heat production and heat loss. Regulation is carried out by physiological mechanisms which can change both heat production and heat loss in an appropriate manner [2].

Nervous System Regulation

The regulation of body temperature occurs in an integration centre situated in the brain, in the hypothalamus. Peripheral heat temperature receptors in the skin and in various other parts of the body send signals concerning ambient temperature to that center.

The somatic sensory area in the cortex also participates in thermoregulation. Sensations of cold and heat transferred to that area enable us to act appropriately (modify behavior) to help control temperature. The somatic area is also connected with the thermoregulation center in the hypothalamus.

The thermoregulation center consists of two parts. The area in the anterior hypothalamus is activated by signals of heat. It is sensitive to core temperature and activates heat loss mechanisms to cool the body down. The posterior part is activated by signals of cold, and activates heat production to warm the body up. These two areas are interconnected.

Information on temperature in various parts of the body, that is required for thermoregulation, is obtained from peripheral and central receptors. The central receptor in the hypothalmus reacts sensitively to changes in core temperature. Whenever necessary, it will send impulses to correct the situation to the integration center. Peripheral thermoreceptors in the skin react to changes in ambient temperature and mediate this information via sensory nerves to the thermoregulation center in the hypothalamus and to the somatic sensory area in the cortex. Any information from the skin will activate the thermoregulation center to a lesser extent than information received via the central receptor from inner parts of the organism [3]. However, the regulation center constantly integrates information from both sources.

Production and Loss of Heat

The body produces heat through metabolism by the metabolic energy transformations. In physical activity, muscle cell metabolism and heat production increase. With exercise, only a small amount of energy is converted to external work (e.g. walking and bicycling). The mechanic efficiency of human metabolism is quite low, maximally 25%. Most, i.e. 75%, of the chemical energy from physical activity is transformed to heat. In maximal physical activity heat production can be increased 10- to 15-fold compared with heat production at rest.

Cell metabolism is regulated by catecholamines from the adrenals and thyroxine (a hormone produced by the thyroid gland). Increased secretion of either intensifies cell metabolism and raises body temperature [4]. Catecholamines exert their effect through the sympathetic part of the autonomic nervous system, and can increase body heat production by 30–50%. The hypothalamus-pituitary system regulates thyroid gland function and thyroxine production. Increased thyroxine production intensifies cell metabolism and may promote heat production to twice the normal level.

During prolonged heavy exercise, increased heat production is compensated for by more effective loss of heat. Body heat is lost through radiation, conduction, convection, and evaporation. The rate of heat loss (fig. 1) depends on the thermal gradient between the skin and the ambient air. a high gradient causes rapid dissipation of heat, and physical performance capacity is relatively unaffected. The height of the thermal gradient and its

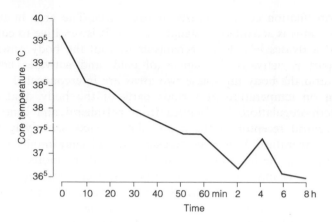

Fig. 1. Restoration of normal core temperature after a cycle race.

stability mainly depend on external circumstances such as temperature, humidity and any movement of air or water. The gradient changes very little especially in dry, moving air.

The main effectors in the heat loss mechanism are the sweat glands and the skin blood flow. Sweating is critical for temperature regulation. If the ambient air is sufficiently dry and moving, any sweat easily evaporates cooling down the surface of the skin. The thermal gradient between skin and ambient air may then either increase or remain stable thus facilitating dissipation of heat [5]. Sweat volume can vary from zero to over 2 liters/h [6]. People acclimatized to hot weather have a higher sweating capacity and can thus dissipate more heat. Sweating is regulated by the hypothalamus through the autonomic cholinergic nervous system, but catecholamines also stimulate sweat glands.

The skin and subcutaneous tissue provide an insulating layer between ambient air and the internal parts of the organism [3]. There is constant blood flow through this insulating layer, and heat is transferred from the body's core via the bloodstream to be evaporated from the skin. Evaporation can be intensified and the insulation capacity and conductance of skin and subcutaneous tissue regulated by enhancing skin circulation. Skin circulation is controlled by the hypothalamus, and orders to increase or to decrease it are mediated by the autonomic nervous system. Skin circulation is also affected by impulses from local receptors in the skin. Its volume can be as high as 30% of cardiac output.

Brown Fat

Brown fat used to be considered as a blood-forming tissue, an organ typical of hibernating species, or as a kind of secretory gland. In the 1960s it was observed to play an important role in regulating body temperature by protecting vital organs against cold.

Brown fat can be found around large vessels such as the carotid arteries, where it serves to raise the temperature of circulating blood. Brown fat is most common in newborn babies, in animals hibernating in cold regions and in people who have lived long enough in a cold climate to become acclimatized. In these groups, brown fat can be found in the back of the shoulders, behind the scapulae where its function is probably to protect the nervous system and the spinal cord [7]. It is activated by sympathetic nerves, which stimulate heat production in the brown fat mitochondria.

The secretion of TSH (thyroid-stimulating hormone) affects the amount of brown fat. An increase in serum TSH level stimulates cell metabolism and the secretion of thyroxine. This in turn raises body temperature. An increase in the amount of brown fat can be observed simultaneously. Both act to keep body temperature normal in a cold environment.

Adaptation to Various Temperatures

Immediate Factors Affecting Performance Capacity in a Hot Climate

When one moves from a cool to a hot climate, heat stress is experienced. The hot environment induces a load on the circulatory system, because the skin blood flow increases for transport of heat for thermoregulatory reasons. This increase in skin blood flow decreases blood flow to the exercising muscles and results in a decreased maximal physical performance capacity. In other words, part of the physical performance capacity must be used to help reduce body temperature [8].

Circulatory Changes. Heart rate increases due to an increased skin circulation and due to a peripheral shift in blood flow to the skin. An increased heart rate and cardiac output intensify cooling of the body. To cool the body down, part of circulating blood is directed to the skin where heat is lost via evaporation of sweat. Skin perfusion may under such circumstances increase by as much as a third of the cardiac output. Simultaneously, the tone of venous capillaries in the skin diminishes leaving plenty of circulating blood in the skin. This, in turn, leads to decreased venous return and to a decline in the amount of blood pumped by the heart each beat [9].

Table 1. Symptoms of dehydration

1	A 1% weight deficit reduces capacity for prolonged exercises
2	A 2% weight deficit (in a man weighing 70 kg, 1.5 litres) causes a feeling of thirst and reduced capacity for physical exercise.
3	A 6% weight deficit (in a man of 70 kg, 4.2 litres) causes feelings of extreme thirst and weakness, irritability, aggression and reduced urinary output; physical and mental performance capacity are decreased
4	A weight deficit exceeding 6% (in a man of 70 kg, more than 4.2 liters) reduces physical and mental performance capacity seriously

Table 2. Symptoms of salt depletion

1	A deficit of 0.5 g/kg (in a man of 70 kg, 35 g) causes fatigue, dizziness, a feeling of weakness and mild muscle twitches.
2	A deficit of 0.5–0.75 g/kg (in a man of 70 kg, 35–52.5 g) causes, in addition to the symptoms listed above, nausea, a feeling of sickness, hypotension, fainting and severe muscle cramps
3	A deficit exceeding 0.75 g/kg (in a man of 70 kg, over 52.5 g) causes loss of initiative, hypotension and loss of consciousness

When blood flow is largely directed to the skin, away from exercising muscles, and cardiac output is reduced, less oxygen is available to the muscles, and their endurance drops [8, 10]. The relative shortage of oxygen in the muscles leads to accumulation of lactic acid at 60% lower workloads ($60\% \dot{V}O_{2max}$) in hot versus cool climates. This lowers the anaerobic threshold and leads to early fatigue during prolonged heavy exercise.

Changes in Distribution of Total Body Water, and Sweating (Table 1). As was stated above, initially changes occur in the distribution of blood flow: due to redistribution of circulation and opening of venous networks, and the central blood volume diminishes. As sweating increases to as high as 1.5 litres/h, plenty of fluid and salts are lost: salt depletion may be as high as 20–25 g daily. Unless this amount of water is replaced by drinking, there will be a significant decrease in circulating blood volume, the heart will pump more weakly, and fatigue/dizziness may occur [11] (table 2).

Metabolic Changes. Exercising under hot conditions raises the body core temperature to higher values than normal. An increase of 1 °C will add cell heat production and oxygen consumption by roughly 13% [12]. Cell metabolism is also stimulated by intensified catecholamine production which is due to the heat stress. Accelerated metabolism needlessly adds to energy consumption and negatively affects performance in endurance events. These changes occur rapidly in response to changing ambient temperatures. No real acclimatization occurs in response to short-term exposure to hot weather, however, few significant changes occur, i.e. in thyroid function.

Long-Term Adaptation to a Hot Climate

When one continues to live and work in a hot climate, changes occur in bodily functions to facilitate coping with heat stress. Such acclimatization improves performance capacity.

Circulatory Changes. As the organism adapts to a hot climate, the body core temperature that was raised initially returns to normal. During this adaptation phase plasma volume is increased. As a result, heart rate and stroke volume at rest and at a certain physical exercise intensity return to their original levels. Cardiac output at rest may be near normal or slightly increased. More blood still flows to the skin than in a cool environment; however, increased sweating rate lowers skin temperature, which reduces the need for skin circulation compared with the situation before acclimatization.

Changes in Distribution of Total Body Water and Sweating. During the first 4–5 days, blood plasma and interstitial fluid volumes increase by 16–20% as a result of fluid and salt retention. This increased plasma volume compensates for the relative plasma hypovolemia due to fluid loss early during the process. During the following 10 days these fluid volumes gradually decrease approaching the values in cool climates [13].

The increased fluid volume results from an increased secretion of antidiuretic hormone (ADH) – central hypovolemia stimulates blood volume receptors. Aldosterone secretion soon increases and sodium retention occurs. The secretion of ADH then falls again.

Metabolic Changes. Thyroid function also gradually decreases and reaches a new steady state level within approximately 2 weeks. Sympatheticotonia returns within 4–5 days to the 'cool' level: this is seen for instance as decreased heart rate. These two changes cause basic cell metabolism and oxygen consumption at rest and during exercise to fall to the cool climate level. Performance capacity thus returns to its normal level as a result of long-term acclimatization [4].

Adaptation to a Cold Climate

In subarctic and mountain areas people are exposed to cold weather routinely. Most of Northern Europe belongs to the subarctic region. Winter sports competitions are arranged either in subarctic or in mountain regions. Adaptation to a cold environment depends on physiological adaptability and on inheritance.

Protective mechanisms enable people to live in unpleasantly cold environments, but what are the physiological reactions against cold? For example cold first changes the electrolyte fluid balance; urinary output increases and some sodium depletion occurs (cf. adaptation to hot environment). This decreases the blood volume, which in turn increases the heart rate even in light physical loading [14]. The reduced blood volume decreases physical performance capacity – a disadvantage in competitive sports. Replenishment of lost electrolytes relatively quickly restores normal fluid and blood volumes. Certain populations, such as the Lapps, have taken salt with their coffee; this may be significant for regulating the electrolyte fluid balance and for maintaining normal physical performance capacity in arctic circumstances.

Factors improving tolerance to cold include peripheral vasoconstriction in the extremities and the skin and enhanced metabolism due to shivering. If the ambient temperature falls below 28 °C, a naked person cannot maintain a normal body temperature at total rest through vasoconstriction only [15]. If the temperature is lower or it is windy, the thermal balance will turn negative unless one puts on clothes or does physical exercise. In people who live chronically in cold climates, vasoconstriction occurs more quickly resulting in greater tolerance to cold temperatures when compared to those staying only temporarily in such climates.

Genetic tolerance to cold may have developed as a result of natural selection because there are clear differences between races. However, genetic changes due to cold are difficult to prove [16]. It seems to be easier to get acclimatized to a hot than to a cold climate. This is probably because humans are a 'tropical species' for whom a cold living environment is foreign. Clothes facilitate adaptation to cold weather. Inherited tolerance to cold is not the same as gradually improved individual tolerance as a result of choice of occupation, training, temporary staying in the cold, or growth, which is a result of physiological adaptation and has little to do with inheritance [15]. Adaptation to cold occurs in children immediately after birth. If a child is born into a cold environment, adaptation to cold occurs naturally during growth. This is assumed also to affect hereditary factors.

It takes about 2–4 weeks for an adult to adapt to cold. This has been confirmed in numerous animal studies. Intermittent exposure to a temperature of −20 °C has been observed to clearly improve tolerance to cold and to decrease tendency to shivering [17]. This suggests that the more often one stays in the cold, the easier it becomes to adapt to it. Even though adaptation to cold is largely dependent on inheritance and body structure, it is also affected by clothing, diet, physical condition and socioeconomic factors.

The effect of hereditary factors and body structure on tolerance to cold was studied in a test including two subject groups [18]. One consisted of

Northern Chinese people who had moved to a warmer region and had not spent time in a cold climate for a long time, and the other one of Southern Chinese people living in a warm area, who had never stayed in a cold region. The test showed that those of Northern Chinese origin were capable of keeping their hand temperature normal in cold water for a longer time. Thus, tolerance to cold would seem to depend, at least to some extent, on hereditary factors. Differences in body structure did not affect tolerance to cold in either group.

Sex

When adaptation of men and women to various weather conditions is compared, it appears that women cope better with the cold and men with the heat [19]. No significant differences have been observed in tolerance to cold between men of various weights. The situation is slightly different for women. Stout, overweight women cope better in the cold than thin women. The subcutaneous isolating layer seems to protect women better than men.

Difference in tolerance to cold between women and men probably depends on differences in how heat is produced and in rates of heat production [20]. For such differences fat tissue is important. The reason why women cope better in the cold than men may be that the metabolic rate in fat tissue is lower in women.

Fat and thin people react differently to changes in ambient temperature. Metabolism is accelerated when the weather gets colder. Increased metabolism results in higher skin and core temperatures. In the cold, metabolism increases more in thin than in fat people. There is an explanation to this: in fat people, the subcutaneous fat layer insulates more effectively from cold weather, and a relatively small increase in heat production is therefore sufficient to keep body temperature normal. Thin people must compensate for the absent insulating layer by enhancing metabolism and heat production to a greater extent. Therefore, fat people suffer less from cold.

Differences between men and women in reaction to cold are measurable in children. These differences are seen more clearly with transient exposure to cold and humidity such as when falling into cold water than with exposure to cold air. This has also been studied in swimmers. In cold water, body temperature falls more rapidly in boys than in girls. A difference is also observable between thin and fat boys, i.e. thin boys lose heat more rapidly in cold water. This depends on the protective effect of a subcutaneous fat layer [17]. Girls usually have more subcutaneous fat than boys.

Physical Training.

Good physical fitness improves the ability to adapt to changing climate and weather conditions and thus promotes the ability to tolerate changes in climate [21]. Tolerance to climatic changes may be a problem for seamen, for instance. Athletes normally living in a warm climate who are in good physical condition have no problem in adapting to subarctic conditions relatively quickly.

Several experiments have been made concerning the dependence between physical fitness and adaptation to cold. In one experiment a group lived for a while in a mountainous area to see how chronic exposure to cold and physical training would affect tolerance to cold. The group was divided into two. One spent its nights in normal warm rooms. The other group slept in quarters with temperatures close to zero. Both groups slept in only their underwear, covered with a blanket. In the daytime, both trained according to a programme devised in advance, directed by a physical education teacher. When tolerance to cold was studied after 5 weeks, it was observed that all slept better in a temperature near to zero than in the beginning of the experiment. It was concluded that the ability to cope in a cold environment improved together with physical fitness. It was also observed that sweating occurred in the cold even though it had the unfavorable effect of further lowering skin and body temperature [21].

One study on seamen was performed to see how a simple gymnastics programme would affect the ability to tolerate frequent changes in environmental temperature. Three groups were formed of sea cadets at the beginning of a cruise: one performed once or twice a week an extra 15–20-min gymnastics programme which was extremely strenuous. The other two groups followed their ordinary fitness programme.

The physical performance capacity of the group with the extra gymnastics programme was clearly better than that in the other two groups throughout the cruise. Working efficiency in the two control groups was best in cool and worst in hot weather. In the group of cadets undergoing the extra gymnastics programme no such differences were observed: their working efficiency remained stable throughout the cruise regardless of changes in temperature and climate [22].

It appears that brief periods of physical training are sufficient to maintain performance capacity in extreme weather where changes in temperature otherwise could cause problems.

Metabolism. Man is relatively poorly equipped to live at low temperatures because we cannot adapt quickly to cold environment by increasing our rate of metabolism. However, clothing and heat produced by physical exercise can help to maintain normal body temperature even under very cold circumstances [23]. In addition, the temperature in peripheral parts of the body can be regulated through vasoconstriction. Peripheral circulation remains clearly more stable in the cold in Eskimos and in professional fishermen than in other people. Eskimos and professional fishermen can maintain a higher finger temperature in ice-cold water than other people [14]. This is of decisive importance for the trade and for survival.

People living in a cold region have been shown to have a higher rate of metabolism than those living in a warm area. Energy consumption is higher in people doing physical exercise in the north than in those doing similar work in the south. Eskimos have a 15–30% higher rate of basic metabolism than people living in a warmer climate. The rate of basic metabolism seems to follow a seasonal rhythm, to some extent [24]. Other people living in similar circumstances as Eskimos also have a higher basic rate of metabolism. Increased basic metabolism seems to be caused mainly by the cold environment because winter and continuous darkness as such cause mental fatigue and physical inactivity which should reduce metabolism [25].

In an animal test, cold was observed to be able to change the ratio between slow-twitch (red) and fast twitch (white) muscle fibres. Adaptation to cold causes a relative decrease in the number of endurable muscle fibres and a relative increase in the number of intermediary (between rapid and slow twitching) muscle fibres. The changes occur in the relative proportion of muscle fibres, not in their absolute number [26].

Effect of Ambient Temperature in Competitive Sports

Hot Climate. The greatest disadvantages for athletes not used to a hot climate are fluid and electrolyte loss through sweating and the resulting fatigue and risk of heat stroke. Nevertheless, sweating is part of the heat regulation system and absolutely necessary. Under normal circumstances, sweating is an advantage because it eliminates heat that is constantly produced with physical exercise and, therefore, prevents 'overheating' of the body [27] (table 3).

Acclimatization to a hot climate significantly increases performance capacity under such conditions. Acclimatization need not wait until the athletes arrive in the hot area. Nearly complete acclimatization can be

Table 3. Basic rules to prevent electrolyte and fluid depletion in endurance events in a hot climate

1	Athletes should be weighed every morning, especially if there is fatigue, irritability, headache or a feeling of weakness
2	Urinary salt or sodium chloride concentration should be determined every week
3	If food does not contain more salt than usual, one should add it
4	Athletes should be encouraged to drink regularly; if one drinks only when thirsty, one gets only about half the amount of fluid required; the feeling of thirst does not correlate with salt depletion in any way: one must therefore drink during training even when not thirsty; 'compulsory drinking' is recommended

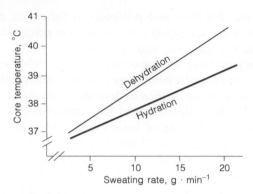

Fig. 2. The relations between sweating rate, fluid balance and core temperature. In dehydration, there is less sweating at an equivalent core temperature than in completely hydrated subjects, and this decreases cooling of the body.

achieved by exposure to a hot room for about 100 min daily (including 50 min of exercise) for 5 weeks. The acclimatization process is very rapid initially with more than 50% occurring during the first 5 days. For reasons of health, alone, such training is absolutely necessary in preparation for competitions in hot environments.

Sufficient acclimatization to a hot climate requires about 10 days in the area. It can be notably delayed by a difference in time. Adaptation can be speeded up by starting acclimatization even before travelling. One can train for some time every day for instance in a warm sauna or in a climate chamber. This will reduce the disadvantages of fluid and electrolyte loss and significantly improve performance.

An athlete travelling to a hot climate must drink copious amounts of fluid, even more than he/she feels necessary, to prevent fluid loss and the resulting fatigue [28, 29]. Cool beverages are more palatable and also help reduce the high temperatures observed during physical exercises. Abundant drinking as such has been enough at rest to reduce core temperature from 39.9 to 39.1 °C. In normal living conditions in hot environment, especially before acclimatization, and during physical exercises it is best to drink more often than normally but only small amounts at one time (fig. 2).

Each year, several athletes worldwide die of heat stroke. Environmental heat illness is the result of a failure of the body's homeostatic mechanism to adequately dissipate an excessive exogenous or endogenous thermal load. The three commonly recognized forms of environmental heat illness are heat cramps, heat exhaustion, and heat stroke. Serious heat illness is most likely to occur either in elderly, inactive people who have decreased capacity to accommodate to environmental heat, or in active young adults such as athletes or military recruits in whom increased endogenous generation of heat through physical activity combines with increased environmental heat exposure.

Intensive physical activity for only 5 min may raise body temperature to 39 °C, and such activity for 10 min may get it up to 40 °C. A hot and humid climate is disadvantageous especially for participants in endurance events because evaporation of sweat drastically reduces; when in a hot humid environment, sweat no longer evaporates but remains on the skin. When this occurs, heat is no longer dissipated and body temperature starts to increase. The final outcome is heat stroke. Heat stroke is a severe, acute disease which is due to disturbance of enzymatic reactions and to instability of the heat regulation system. It can be prevented by wearing suitable clothing permeable to heat and by drinking and eating sufficiently before, during and after competition. Cool showers can be taken during competition. Rapid cooling of the body by, e.g. cold shower is effective as first aid [30]. In more severe cases, intraveneous fluids are required, and unconscious patients must be hospitalized immediately.

Even though sweating helps maintain temperature in high environmental temperatures, excessive sweat loss negatively affects physical performance capacity. Abundant sweating decreases the circulating fluid volume, or blood volume, increasing the work load on the heart. In sweat, electrolytes are lost including sodium, chloride and potassium, which are important for the maintenance of fluid balance. In a hot climate, salt loss may first be excessive (roughly 20 g/day) but it decreases later after complete acclimatization, i.e. after 4–6 weeks, to 3–5 g/day.

Maximal sweating capacity increases during the first 10 days. As a result of acclimatization, sweating starts more easily and at a lower physical exercise intensity than in a cold climate. After acclimatization, sweat production is still higher than in a cool climate but sweat contains less salts. As a result of acclimatization, reuptake of salt in the organism and resistance to salt loss become more intensive.

The organism first strives to reduce fluid loss by increasing the secretion of antidiuretic hormone (ADH). ADH reduces fluid excretion via the kidneys. Aldosterone hormone secretion subsequently also increases and, as a result, sodium is no longer excreted. The secretion of ADH then falls back to the normal level.

Unconsciousness due to severe salt depletion can be differentiated from heat stroke by measuring rectal temperature and determining salt content in the urine. If the rectal temperature is unusually high, the patient suffers from heat stroke. Measures must then be immediately taken to lower the patient's body temperature.

Salt depletion during prolonged exercises causes fatigue, irritability

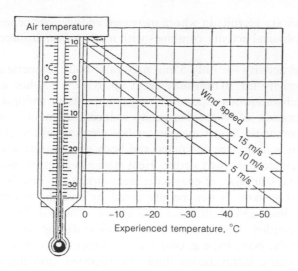

Air temperature

Wind speed

15 m/s
10 m/s
5 m/s

Experienced temperature, °C

Fig. 3. Wind increases the 'frost effect' of cold air. If the temperature is 0 °C and wind speed 10 m/s, the 'frost effect' is similar to that of a temperature of −15 °C in calm weather (Eriksson et al. 1985).

and muscle cramps. Drinks with no salt should not be taken in abundance to replace fluid lost in physical exercises, sport competitions and prolonged performances because such fluids are not retained in the body. Saltless fluids are excreted nearly immediately via the kidneys as urine. Salts retain fluid in the body. Mineral waters and other beverages containing salt are useful for the maintenance of fluid electrolyte balance.

Cold Climate. For athletes living in a subarctic area cold weather is the problem. This is generally less problematic than a hot climate because it is easier to protect oneself against cold than against heat. Disadvantages of cold weather include frostbite, common colds, respiratory symptoms and an increased need for food due to increased basal metabolism, which may be disregarded. In a cold and humid climate breathing might be unpleasant leading to lack of oxygen in the tissues, fatigue, and, in sports events, surprising interruptions may occur. Complete acclimatization to both a cold and a hot climate takes several weeks. General and local (peripheral) tolerance to cold increases as a result of acclimatization.

Frostbite is due to intensive constriction of superficial blood vessels; this is – contrary to what occurs in hot weather – due to the body's trying to preserve all possible heat. When superficial circulation ceases, frostbite results. If the tissue freezes, it becomes necrotic. Frostbite sometimes occurs in skiers' fingers if they wear gloves of a poor quality, even though circulation in the fingers generally remains normal for as long as possible (fig. 3).

Exercising in cold weather is normally not detrimental for health. However, jogging and training in a temperature below −20 °C may be dangerous. For instance accidental loss of mobility may, in a sparsely inhabited area, lead to freezing to death. In temperatures below zero, special attention must be paid to clothing. Training outfits must be warm. Wearing several cloth layers is recommended. Air is trapped between the layers and keeps one warm better than a thick sweater.

If training is intensive from the beginning, 15 min of proper warming up is apt to eliminate increased muscle tonus and stiffness due to cold. Warm up increases muscle temperature and prevents strains and pains. It is easy to catch a cold if one rests in between training or moves very little. Cold weather will not harm the lungs of a healthy person, even though breathing of air with a temperature below zero may feel unpleasant. Before getting to pulmonary alveoli inhaled air reaches the body temperature. In individuals with asthma breathing of cold air can increase the susceptibility to asthmatic attacks.

Breathing in cold weather can be made more pleasant by wearing a mask warming up the air to be inhaled. Such a mask works well in light training of, for example, running or skiing, but in hard training with increased breath rate resistance to air flow greatly increases and breathing through the mask may feel laborious. Such a mask can also be used to increase the strength of breathing muscles, if for nothing else.

Adaptation to Time Changes

Circadian Rhythms and Jet Lag

The human body follows a regular rhythm of roughly 24 h, a 'circadian rhythm'. It is primarily regulated by the suprachiasmatic nuclei in the hypophysis. Another important human rhythm is the 25- to 35-day monthly rhythm [31]. If one crosses several (more than four) time zones within only a few hours, jet lag will occur resulting in overwhelming fatigue and decreased physical performance capacity. Jet lag occurs because the biological clock has not had time to adjust to the local time [32]. Moreover, before acclimatization there is dysrhythmia between biological and social daily rhythms such as working, training and resting patterns.

Body temperature, performance capacity and secretion of most hormones, related to metabolism such as cortisol and melatonin secretion, depending on changes in light, follow circadian rhythms [33, 34]. When the daily rhythm is disturbed, changes of temperature and cortisol secretion return to normal more slowly than the sleep–awake pattern.

Table 4. Buley's formula [35]

$$\frac{\text{Travel hours}}{2} + Z_{\text{diff}} > 4 + C_d + C_a = 10(\text{days rest})$$

Local time	C_d	C_a
08.00–11.59	0	4
12.00–17.59	1	2
18.00–21.59	3	0
22.00–00.59	4	1
01.00–07.59	3	3

This formula, devised by the late Dr. Buley, formerly of ICAO, in 1967, is intended for use by air travellers but is not suitable for flight crews. As an example a passenger travelling from London to Los Angeles, with an 8-hour time-zone change, leaving at 18.00 h LT and arriving at 21.00 h LT requires $\frac{11}{2} + (8 - 4) + 3 + 0$ tenths of a day free = 1.25 days, and this is then rounded up to the next $\frac{1}{2}$ day = 1.5 days (ICAO).

Most bodily functions are most active in the afternoon and least active after midnight. The circadian rhythm could in principle be largely regulated with light. The secretion of melatonin and cortisol is greatest when there is less light, i.e. at night and early in the morning. Light prevents melatonin secretion from the pineal body. Melatonin affects the biological clock. It is possible to reduce jet lag by taking melatonin on several consecutive days.

After flights crossing several time zones circadian rhythms fall out of phase with the local time. Adaptation to the difference depends on the number of time zones crossed, flight direction, flight time and individual factors. As a rule of thumb, adaptation to a new daily rhythm requires as many days as the time difference is in hours. This is, however, not the same as estimated by Buley's formula (table 4).

When flying east (phase difference forward) adaptation takes longer than when flying west (phase difference backward). It is evidently easier to lengthen than to shorten the daily rhythm. When one flies west, the circadian rhythms become longer and it is easier to adapt to the change. When one flies east, the rhythms become shorter, causing greater adaptation problems. The biological clock should be decelerated when flying west and accelerated when flying east. This can occur artificially with some drugs. Lithium and alcohol slow down the inner pacemaker of sleep-awake pattern and tricyclic antidepressants acclerate it. Therefore, alcohol can be used flying west, but not east.

Restoration of a normal daily rhythm (sleep-wake pattern) occurs more rapidly than complete adaptation (hormonal secretion and diurnal body temperature changes) to the new time zone. If one for instance crosses seven time zones west, restoration of normal sleep-wake rhythm takes about 3 days but complete adaptation to the new time zone some 6 days.

It has been estimated that about every fourth air passenger has practically no problem in adapting to the time difference. These lucky people find the new rhythm quickly after the flight. In some, however, flying causes difficult symptoms. Adaptation is also affected by age: old people adapt more slowly to the new time than younger ones. Delayed adaptation frequently occurs in people over the age of 40. Way of life also affects adaptation. People working in the evening usually find it easier to adapt to time differences [36].

Ways to Promote Adaptation

Both mental performance capacity and physical performance capacity can be decreased by an average of 1–3% after a medium-distance flight crossing time zones, but sometimes by as much as 8–12%. This corresponds to mild intoxication. Both brain function and nerve-muscle coordination are impaired which means that this phenomenon is significant especially in competitive sports. In athletes, concentration is often disturbed by discontinuous sleep and early morning awakening after flights across several time zones. Sleep disturbances are usually greatest approximately 2 days after a flight when fatigue due to staying awake has disappeared and some acclimatization has occurred.

If the phase difference forward (eastward) is for instance 12 h, the athlete should travel to the site of competition a fortnight in advance to allow for a sufficiently long time of acclimatization. Differences in temperature (heat or cold) may further lengthen the time required for acclimatization.

Adaptation can be enhanced and jet lag reduced by the following:

(1) Daytime flights.

(2) After reaching the destination, slight exercise before going to bed will reduce interruptions of sleep; restrict alcoholic drinks, coffee and smoking because they increase such interruptions.

(3) Falling asleep is facilitated by eating carbohydrates, staying awake by food rich in proteins. It is useful to drink plenty of soft drinks and juices during the flight, but sleeping pills should be avoided.

(4) Adjusting one's bedtime or the time of getting up back or forth before the flight may be useful. If possible, one should go to bed 1 to 2 h later (when travelling west) or earlier (when travelling east) on a couple of nights before the flight.

(5) On board the plane, one should adjust one's watch immediately to the new time. When reaching the destination, habits should be immediately

changed to accord with the new time: one should sleep at night and stay awake during the day.

(6) The local rhythm of life should be adopted at once. If it is absolutely necessary to take a nap during the daytime, it should be done between noon and 5 p.m. Such a nap should not take more than 2 h.

(7) One should spend as much time as possible out in the sun. Evening light when flying west, and morning light when flying east, promote adaptation. After flying east, one should not sleep too long in the morning.

Conclusion

People normally living in a cool climate perform more poorly in heavy exercise when the weather is suddenly warm. In principle, performance capacity also decreases when one moves rapidly from a hot to a cold or cool climate. Acclimatization to a hot climate significantly increases performance capacity under such conditions. Acclimatization need not wait until the athletes arrive in the hot area. Nearly complete acclimatization can be achieved by exposure to a hot room for about 100 min daily (including 50 min of exercise) for 5 weeks. An athlete travelling to a hot climate must drink copious amounts of fluid, even he/she feels necessary, to prevent fluid loss and the resulting fatigue. Cool beverages are more palatable and also help reduce the high temperatures observed during physical exercise. For athletes living in a subarctic area cold weather is the problem. This is generally less problematic than hot weather because it is easier to protect oneself against cold than against heat. Complete acclimatization to both a cold and a hot climate takes several weeks. After flights crossing several time zones circadian rhythms fall out of phase with the local time. Adaptation to the difference depends on the number of time zones crossed, flight direction, flight time and individual factors. As a rule of thumb, adaptation to a new daily rhythm requires as many days as the time difference is in hours.

References

1   Garden JW, Wilson JD, Rash PJ: Acclimatization of healthy young adult males to hot-wet environment. J Appl Physiol 1966;21:655–669.
2   Randall WC, Rawson RO, McCook RD, Peiss CN: Central and peripheral factors in dynamic thermoregulations. J Appl Physiol 1963;18:61–64.
3   Wyndham CH: Role of skin and core temperatures in man's temperature regulation. J Appl Physiol 1965;20:31–36.
4   Sellers EA, Flattery KV, Shuh A, Johnson GE: Thyroid status in relation to catecholamines in cold and warm environments. Can J Physiol Pharmacol 1971;49:268–275.

5   Kraning II KK, Belding HS, Hertig BA: Use of sweating rate to predict other physiological responses to heat. J Appl Physiol 1966;21:111–117.

6   Maugham RJ: Fluid and electrolyte loss and replacement in exercise. J Sports Sci 1991;9:117–142.

7   Doniach D: Possible stimulation of thermogenesis in brown adipose tissue by thyroid-stimulating hormone. Lancet 1975;ii:7926:160–161.

8   Nielsen B: Heat stress causes fatigue! Exercise performance during acute and repeated exposure to hot, dry environments. Med Sport Sci 1991;in press.

9   Rowell LB, Kraning II KK, Kennedy JW, Evans TO: Central circulatory responses to work in dry heat before and after acclimatization. J Appl Physiol 1967;22:509–518.

10 Nielsen B, Savard G, Richter EA, Hargreaves M, Saltin B: Muscle blood flow and muscle metabolism during exercise and heat stress. J Appl Physiol 1990;69:1040–1046.

11 Wyndham CH, Benade AJA, Williams CG, Strydom NB, Goldin A, Heyns AJA: Changes in central circulation and body fluid spaces during acclimatization to heat. J Appl Physiol 1965;20:37–45.

12 Karvonen J: Warming-up and its physiological effects. Acta Univ Ouluensis Pharm Physiol 1978;30:1–50.

13 Marcus P: Heat acclimatization by exercise-induced elevation of body temperature. J Appl Physiol 1972;33:283–288.

14 Liakh LA: Effect of body temperature on biochemical changes in the blood during cold adaption. Fiziol Zh 1976;62:294–303.

15 Slonim AD, Shevetsova EJ: Chemical thermoregulation after accelerated adaption to cold. Fiziol Zh 1973;59:1262–1267.

16 Kamon E: Ergonomics of heat and cold. Texas Rep Biol Med 1975;33:145–185.

17 Sloan RE, Keatinge WR: Cooling rates of young people swimming in cold water. J Appl Physiol 1973;35:371–373.

18 So JK: Genetic, acclimatizational and anthropometric factors in hand cooling among North and South Chinese. Am J Phys Anthrop 1975;43:31–38.

19 Jones RE, Little MA, Thomas RB, Hoff CJ, Dufour DL: Local cold exposure on Andean indians during normal and simulated activities. Am J Phys Anthrop 1976;44:305–313.

20 Hadland DG, Stock JF: Heat and cold tolerance. Relation to body weight. Postgrad Med 1974;55:75–80.

21 Karvonen J: Die Wirkung des kalten Klimas auf den Organismus und das Leistungsvermögen. Med Sport 1975;15:56–57.

22 Hellström R, Lindroth K: Physical working capacity, training and climate. Acta Med Scand 1967;472:207.

23 Nadel RE, Holmer J, Bergh U, Åstrand PO, Stolwijk JAJ: Thermoregulatory shivering during exercise. Life Sci 1973;13:983–989.

24 Sjöstrand T: Clinical Physiology. Stockholm, Victor Petterssons Bokindustri, 1967, p 1971.

25 Tikhomirov JJ: The nature of metabolic processes in polar exposures. Noprosy pitanija 1973;32:37–40.

26 Beribas VI, Filiptchenko RE: The morphofunctional changes in the muscle fibres after the cold adaption and muscular activity. Fiziol Zh 1974;60:566–575.

27 Libert JP, Amros C, Di Nisi J, Muzet A, Fukuda H, Ehrhart J: Thermoregulatory adjustments during continuous heat exposure. Eur J Appl Physiol 1988;57:499–506.

28 Nielsen B: Dehydration, rehydration and thermoregulation. Med Sport Sci 1984;17:81–96.

29 Nielsen B: Effects of fluid ingestion on heat tolerance and exercise performance; in Hales

JRS, Richards DAB (eds): Heat Stress, Physical Exertion and Environment. Amsterdam, Elsevier, 1987, pp 1–13.

30   Pandolf KB, Cadarette BS, Sawka MN, Young AJ, Francesconi RP, Conzales RR: Thermoregulatory responses of middle-aged and young men during dry-heat acclimation. J Appl Physiol 1988;85:65–71.

31   Karvonen J: Medicine in Sports. Kuopio, Publications of the University of Kuopio, 1990, p 34.

32   Stein JH: Disorders in sleep-wake cycle; in Stein JH (ed): Internal Medicine. Boston, Little, Brown, 1990, p 1910.

33   Härmä M: Kolmivuorotyötä tekevän henkilökunnan terveys, fyysinen suorituskyky ja vuorotyöhön sopeutuminen. Kuopio, Publications of the University of Kuopio, 1985, pp 14–25.

34   Aschoff J, Wever R: Über Reproduzierbarkeit circadianer Rhythmen beim Menschen. Klin Wochenschr 1980;58:323–335.

35   Buley LE: Experience with a physiologically based formula on determining rest periods on long distance air travel. Aerospace Med 1970;41:680.

36   Plett R, Colquhoun WP, Condon R, Knauth P, Rutenfranz J, Eickhoff S: Work at sea: A study of sleep, and of circadian rhythms in physiological functions, in watchkeepers on merchant vessels. Int Arch Occup Environ Health 1988;60:395–403.

Dr. Juha Karvonen, National Agency for Welfare and Health,
P.O. Box 220, SF-00531 Helsinki (Finland)

Karvonen J, Lemon PWR, Iliev I (eds): Medicine in Sports Training and Coaching.
Med Sport Sci. Basel, Karger, 1992, vol 35, pp 69–103

Training at Altitude

Ilcho Iliev

National Academy of Sports, Sofia, Bulgaria

Contents

Introduction

The problems of altitude training are relatively new ones. Thirty years ago, during the Rome Olympics, when a runner from Ethiopia, Abebe Bikila, surprisingly won the marathon race only a few specialists mentioned that he was born and trained at an altitude of 2,000–2,500 m above sea level. At that time the effects of medium altitude on exercise capacity and sport performances were largely unknown. Several years later, when Mexico City was selected as the site of the 1968 Olympic games it was suddenly realized, how little was known about the limitations for sport performance and training at altitudes close to 2,300 m.

As a consequence, in a very short period of time many research groups all over the world studied the most important practical aspects of acclimatization and training at altitudes close to 2,300 m.

National and international symposia were held in Alma Ata, 1965, [1] Milan, 1966 [2], Albuquerque, 1966 [3], Magglingen, 1966 [4], and Moscow, 1966 [5], 1967 [6]. Numerous publications in international journals appeared in the period 1965–1968, devoted to the scientific and practical problems of training and performing at medium altitude (in the range 1,800–3,400 m). The results of this extremely intensive research, though not without some controversies in details, served as the basis for reasonable practical recommendations concerning acclimatization and training at altitude for the competitors of the Mexico Olympics.

The Olympic competitions, although not a strictly controlled experiment provided a verification for most of the available scientific knowledge on the physical and physiological bases of sport performance at medium altitude. Briefly, this can be summarized as follows: after acclimatization and training of 2–3 weeks at altitude, sport performances which depend on speed and power might be slightly better, but all events depending on endurance would be adversely affected in proportion to the duration of the respective activity [7]. As expected, the hypoxic handicap was more severe for athletes originating from sea level regions, than for those, born and trained at higher altitudes. In the final of the 10,000 m race, 5 of the first 6 places were occupied by athletes native to high altitude or domiciled there for a prolonged period. However, the time of the winner, Naftali Temu of Kenya (29 min 27.4 s) was almost 2 min slower than the world record set in 1965 by Ron Clark. Incidentally, Clark finished sixth in Mexico in a state of collapse and had to recover under the administration of oxygen [8].

It should be mentioned, however, that as a 'side effect' of the altitude training, used by some athletes in preparation for the Mexico Olympic Games a series of world class performances were set a short time before and immediately after the 1968 Olympics. For example, following consecutive 2 or 3 weeks training camps at altitude Jim Ryan set up world records at sea level in the mile (3.51.3) and in the 1,500 m (3.33.1). Five of six world class athletes, who trained together with him also produced best personal performances in middle distance events [9]. The Bulgarian athlete Michail Jelev, using prolonged altitude training in the period 1967–1969 improved the national record for 3,000 m steplechase four times (from a very mediocre 8.41.4 to an excellent for that epoch 8.25.0).

The scientific reasons for this and other excellent athletic performances at sea level after altitude training was the topic of a joint meeting of the British Association of Sport and Medicine and the British Olympic Association held in London in 1973. Unfortunately, the papers presented on this meeting did not allow a definitive conclusion as to whether altitude training itself or other factors improved performance after coming down from altitude training camps.

Nevertheless, the interest in the potential benefits of altitude training was not lost and, though not so intensive, research was continued on acclimatization and training at altitude and on the reacclimatization after returning to a normal environment. During the past decade several excellent performances of world-class athletes were achieved after altitude training. Nicolina Shtereva won gold medals in the 800 m race at the European Cup in Milan in July 1979 and at the World Cup in Montreal in September 1979. Totka Petrova finished first in the 1,500 m race in Milan 1979 and produced the best world performance (3.57.4) during the Balkan Games in the same year. Both trained for 3–4 weeks in June and in August at a training camp on Belmeken, in Rila Mountain, 2,050 m above sea level [Bonov, chief coach of middle and long distance runners, personal commun.].

Between 1982 and 1984, the female team of the German middle distance runners trained in Saint Moritz, at an altitude of 1,900 m, and set German records and personal best performances afterwards winning two medals (silver and bronze) and three fourth places in the European and World championships [10]. The famous Norwegian runner Ingrid Kristiansen set her 1985 world record in the 10,000 m (30.59.42) after training in Saint Moritz as well [10]. Sigrun Wodars won the Olympic 800 m race in Seoul, September 1988, after training camps at altitude in July (Mexico) and August (Belmeken) [Bonov, personal commun.].

The swimmers of former DDR routinely held training camps at altitudes between 1,800 and 2,800 m for many years and have regularly shown excellent, world-class performances [11]. Also German rowing teams have successfully used altitude training for improving $\dot{V}O_2$ max and endurance capacity of competitors before important championships [12].

So despite the lack of unequivocal scientific evidence of the benefits of altitude training, it is used by many coaches aiming to increase endurance performance of elite athletes.

The aim of the following review is to present the physiological rationale of altitude training and to discuss some practical aspects of coaching during the most delicate periods of acclimatization at altitude and the reacclimatization after returning from altitude camps.

Physiological Background

The major physiologically important characteristic of the altitude environment is the lower than sea level barometric pressure and, as a consequence, the lower partial pressure of oxygen. Other characteristics of smaller, if not negligible importance are the lower mean temperatures, the broader range of day to night and of sunlight to shadow temperatures, the lower relative humidity of air, the higher solar radiation, and the increased ionisation of air.

Barometric Pressure and Partial Pressure of Oxygen

Barometric pressure (PB) is an exponential function of altitude which, from sea level to an altitude of 8,500 m, may be approximately described by the following, empirically derived equation:

$$PPB = 864.4 \cdot \exp(-0.1058 \, A) - 104,$$

where PB = barometric pressure (mm Hg) and A = altitude (km).

The graph of the above function is presented in figure 1. Actual PB may vary slightly from the calculated values during different seasons and/or at different geographic zones. However, the differences are small and only of physiological importance at very high altitudes, where even small changes may create dramatic consequences for the homeostasis of the organism.

The partial pressure of oxygen in the inspired air, after its saturation with water vapour in the trachea may be expressed as a function of altitude by the equation:

$$pO_2 = 181 \cdot \exp(-0.1051 \, A) - 32.2,$$

where pO_2 = partial pressure of oxygen = 0.2094(PB-47), and A = altitude (km). The graph of this function is presented by the upper curve in figure 2.

At sea level the mean alveolar pressure of oxygen (pAO_2) is about 50 mm lower than the tracheal pO_2. Consequently, a similar curve, representing pAO_2 as a function of altitude would be expected. However, because of the adaptive increase of lung ventilation at altitude, the slope of the pAO_2 curve, as presented by the lower curve on figure 2, is less than that of the pO_2 curve in tracheal air. The respective equation is:

$$pAO_2 = 100.4 \cdot \exp(-0.1548 \, A).$$

Actual pAO_2 values may differ slightly from those predicted by the above equation because of environmental factors, individual variability of breathing pattern, or other physiological reasons, but as mentioned above the respective differences are generally small and may be neglected in most cases, when discussing altitudes near to 2,000 m.

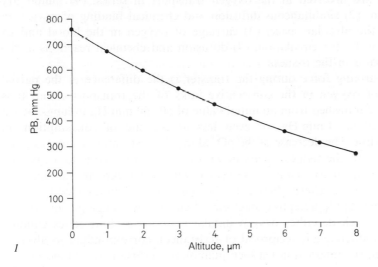

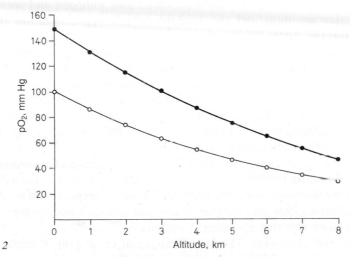

Fig. 1. Barometric pressure as a function of altitude.

Fig. 2. Parial pressure of oxygen in tracheal air (upper curve) and in alveolar air (lower curve) as a function of altitude.

Physiological Consequences of the Decreased pAO_2

It is well known that the human organism is dependent on oxygen. If the required oxygen consumption for the normal function of the living body is to be maintained, an equivalent flow of oxygen has to be supplied from the ambient air to the sites of utilisation. Various systems and functions are involved in the oxygen transport in series: (1) pulmonary ventilation; (2) simultaneous diffusion and chemical binding of oxygen in blood in the alveolar space; (3) carriage of oxygen in the blood and its distribution by the circulation; (4) diffusion and chemical reactions in the mitochondria in the tissues.

The driving force during the transfer is the difference in the partial pressure of oxygen in the consecutive links of the transport chain. It is gradually diminished from an initial value of 50–60 mm Hg in lungs, at sea level, to about 1 mm Hg, or even less at the site of consumption, in mitochondria. The decrease of the pO_2 along the respiratory chain from the inspired air to the tissues occurs in various steps, analogous to a cascade: from ambient air to airway air saturated with water vapour, subsequently to alveolar air to arterial blood, to the cells and to venous blood.

Shephard [13], accepting an electrical current flow analogue derived an equation which describes oxygen uptake in terms of four series conductances (conductance is reciprocal of resistance), corresponding to alveolar ventilation, the interaction between pulmonary diffusion and blood flow in lungs, blood transport, and interaction between tissue diffusion and perfusion. Using this equation and the available physiological data on the behaviour and the limits of the above functions (alveolar ventilation, pulmonary diffusion of oxygen, blood flow and blood transport capacity, tissue diffusion and perfusion) at sea level and at an altitude of 2,300 m, for normal men and for athletes, he calculated that unacclimatized sea level residents will suffer a physiological disadvantage of 4–8% in the endurance events held at altitude. This handicap would be largely reversed by a corresponding increase in the oxygen capacity of the blood. For this to occur, a series of adaptive changes are needed. Unfortunately, none of these are automatically guaranteed even during prolonged acclimatization and training at altitude, because of the interaction of many, partially controversial mechanisms along the chain of oxygen transport system. As a result of acclimatization and training at medium altitudes many adaptive changes have been reported by different authors.

Faulkner and co-workers [14, 15], Weidemann et al. [16], Kurenkov and Absaljamov [17], and Iliev and colleagues [18, 19], observed very small changes in $\dot{V}O_2$ max on arrival at 2,000–2,400 m, while Asahina et al. [20], Volkov et al. [21], and Muchamedjarov [22] described a decrease of $\dot{V}O_2$ max of up to 27–30% as compared to sea level values. Murray et al, [23], using treadmill running in a decompression chamber at a simulated altitude of 2,300 m, found a 23% decrease in $\dot{V}O_2$ max. Farfel et al. [24] found a decrease in $\dot{V}O_2$ max values of 10–18% in athletes of different sports. According to Faulkner et al. [25] $\dot{V}O_2$ max values at altitude where 13% lower, corresponding to a 6% worse performance in a 3-miles trial. Using a decompression chamber (simulated altitude of 2,300 m) Saltin [26] observed a decrease of $\dot{V}O_2$ max of 16%. Similar data were published by Hollmann [27] and Drews [28], both using hypoxic gas mixtures corresponding to an altitude of 2,300 m. Roskamm et al. [29] found a comparable decrease of $\dot{V}O_2$ max (8–14%) during experiments in a low-pressure chamber and during a stay in Mexico City. Similar findings were published by Owen and Pugh [30], who studied elite British athletes in London and in Mexico City, by Bierstecker and van Leeven [31] for Dutch athletes, and by Scano et al. [32] for the Italian participants in the Pre Olympic Games, 1966, in Mexico.

In summary: A decrease of the maximal oxygen uptake at altitude is theoretically expected and is in fact found by many authors, in artificial (laboratory) and in natural environment. The broad range of variability of published experimental data suggest that additional factors may be involved in the results observed at altitude.

The Adaptive Changes Evoked by the Reduced PO_2

If the pO_2 in the inspired air is decreased the organism struggles to maintain the necessary minimal mitochondrial pO_2 by a number of adaptive mechanisms: (1) increased lung ventilation and cardiac output at rest and at any given level of submaximal exercise; (2) readjustment of the regional circulation in the lungs and in the tissues with elevated oxygen demands; (3) increased capillary bed and capillary blood volume in active tissues; (4) slower capillary blood flow in active capillary bed, thus increasing diffusion time along the capillary; (5) increased red cell count and haemoglobin concentration in blood and myoglobin concentration in muscle cells; (6) shift of the oxygen-haemoglobin dissociation curve to the right and elevated levels of 2,3-diphosphoglycerate (2,3-DPG); (7) structural and metabolic adaptations on cellular and subcellular levels (mitochondrial density, enzyme activities, hormonal levels, buffering capacity and others).

Some of the above mechanisms are rapid and are immediately mobilized to minimize hypoxia at tissue level as much as possible. Others are slower and need several days, weeks, or months for maximal efficiency. Some appear to be genetically determined and are very resistant to change.

Increased lung ventilation is obviously one of the most rapid mechanisms to compensate for the lower pO in ambient air. Inasmuch as lower partial pressure of oxygen is equivalent to a smaller number of O_2 molecules in a given volume of air, a simple way to preserve the delivery rate of oxygen is to increase the volume of air entering the lungs at a given time, i.e. the ventilation rate of the alveolar space. Knowing that in the normal population the adaptive range of the respiratory function is extremly wide (1:20, or even more) it may be expected that, at least at rest and during submaximal exercise, when a relatively small part of the whole adaptive capacity has to be mobilized, a perfect compensation might be realized due to the above mechanism. However, it is not this simple, because of the complexity of the oxygen uptake and delivery system. If something happens to any of the constituent links of the chain, adaptive changes are needed all over the system to compensate, or an impairment will result. An increased lung ventilation could be realized through an increase of breathing frequency and/or by expansion of the tidal volume. As a consequence, both alveolar space and alveolar ventilation may be different at seemingly equivalent levels of lung ventilation, according to the breathing pattern. For optimal efficiency, at any given level of alveolar ventilation, adaptive changes of lung circulation and alveolar perfusion are needed, resulting in respective changes of the regional blood pressure and of the active capillary bed in lungs. Expansion of the lung capillary bed increases the blood volume and the contact surface between air and blood in alveolar space, simultaneously slowing blood flow, thus allowing for a longer contact time. As a result a more favourable environment is created for the diffusion and chemical binding of oxygen in blood, even without any shift in the diffusing capacity.

All these changes are adaptive in nature, but in some subjects and under some specific conditions they may have unfavourable consequences as well, leading in extreme cases to high altitude pulmonary edema.

It is of note that the described changes in lung ventilation and perfusion, which may compensate for the lower pO_2 in air and preserve the oxygen delivery rate, have an intrinsic unfavourable side effect, namely they all contribute to a larger than normal washout of CO_2 from venous blood in lungs. The carbon dioxide is an endproduct of oxidative metabolism, which is normally produced in the tissues and eliminated by the lungs at a rate proportional to the metabolic rate, so that its concentration in blood in a normal environment is controlled in a narrow range. But CO_2 is not only a waste product of metabolism, it is also an important ingredient of the acid-base balance of the organism and a specific regulator of the respiratory function. An enhanced washout of CO_2 at altitude, because of the hyperventilation at rest and during exercise is prone to provoke metabolic and respiratory disorders, impairing oxygen transport and utilisation. While normally the hypoxic drive and the CO_2 concentration in blood are additive stimuli for respiration, at altitude they become antagonistic. Consequently, the optimal rate of adaptive hyperventilation at altitude is based on a compromise between hypoxic drive and hypocapnia created by the increased ventilation rate. As a result, non-linear relationships between pAO_2 and lung ventilation are to be expected at altitude, particularly in the earlier phases of acclimatization to the hypoxic environment. During this initial period of functional readjustment, any level of ventilation, in the wide range between hypoventilation and hyperventilation, may occur. This is actually the case, according to published experimental data by different research groups.

Theoretically, at an altitude of 2,300 m an increase of lung ventilation of about 30% is needed for a perfect compensation of the lower pO_2. Practically reported values are in the range from merely 4–6% in decompression chambers at simulated 2,400 m [29], to 56% in the natural environment at similar altitudes [24, 32]. Mostly an increase of 15–20% was found at rest and during submaximal exercise [19, 29, 33]. Similarly, very different values of maximum exercise ventilation were described by different research groups. The published data are in the range from no change [34, 37], or a minimal increase [15], through 15–25% [18, 26, 27, 38, 39] to an increase of 59% [32]. The extremely wide range of data, published by different research groups may be due to several possibilities. These include experimental design (low pressure chambers, hypoxic gas mixtures, or natural environment at different altitudes), the work loads (laboratory tests or athletic trials with different intensity and/or duration), the subjects (trained, untrained, with or without previous altitude experience, different sex and age), or some other physiological or psychological factors out of research control. Theoretically, slightly higher values of maximum exercise ventilation at altitude, as compared to sea level, might be expected, even without the need for compensation of the lower pO_2, due to the lower density of inspired air and hence lower resistance to the air flow in the lung airways and in the respective tubing in the measuring equipment.

Plausible explanations could be suggested for the observed discrepancies, but the important point in the context of altitude training is that they do really exist. The extremely high dispersion of the published results of strictly controlled experiments suggest that even greater variability may be expected in the field when athletes and coaches go to altitude.

Summarizing the theoretical considerations and the available experimental data on the adaptive changes of lung ventilation and circulation immediately after arriving at altitude, it may be concluded that a perfect compensation for the impairment of the oxygen uptake in lungs is not attainable. So the blood leaving the pulmonary circulation may not be fully saturated with oxygen, which means a smaller transport capacity of the blood will exist at any comparable level of blood volume and/or flow. If at a given level of circulating blood volume the oxygen content of a unit of blood is lower than normal, the only possibility to preserve the oxygen delivery rate to the tissues is to speed up the turnover of the available blood volume, i.e. to increase the circulation rate. This is possible at rest and during submaximal exercise by mobilizing the spare potential of the heart rate, or of the stroke volume of the heart, or both, but obviously it is impossible to increase the maximal cardiac output imposed by the maximal values of the heart rate and the stroke volume.

An increase of the submaximal heart rate and cardiac output during prolonged exercise with moderate intensity at altitudes near to 2,300 m is described by many authors [19, 34, 35, 40, 47]. Maximal heart rate and cardiac output, on the contrary, do not change at moderate altitudes [19, 26, 29, 34, 35, 42, 48, 50]. However, at higher places (3, 500 m and over) they tend to decrease, thus becoming one of the limiting factors of the oxygen transport [40, 44, 51, 54].

The above mechanisms of adaptation, immediately mobilized in the struggle for oxygen, are not the only physiological response to altitude. Further and very important features of the adaptation to the hypoxic environment, which have not been discussed until now are the mechanisms involved in the binding and releasing of oxygen and the oxygen-carrying capacity of the blood. It is well know that oxygen is transported in the blood chemically bound to haemoglobin. The affinity of haemoglobin to oxygen is variable depending on partial pressures of blood gases, pH, temperature and other variables, so that at different sites of circulation the ratio of oxyhaemoglobin to reduced haemoglobin varies. The quantity of oxygen in the blood at a given level of pO_2 in air, of lung ventilation and circulation depends on the concentration of haemoglobin, which is normally proportional to the red cell count. The oxygen supply to the tissues may be described by the following formula:

Oxygen supply (ml/min) = cardiac output (litres/min) · haemoglobin concentration (g/l) · 1.34 (ml O_2/g Hb) · oxygen saturation of haemoglobin,

where saturation is the fraction of haemoglobin molecules containing bound oxygen (HbO_2/Hb total).

Haemoglobin concentration and saturation may change independently. Haemoglobin concentration is a more conservative parameter which needs more time to change, while haemoglobin saturation can change rapidly depending mainly on the pO_2 in blood. Inasmuch as pO_2 varies along the blood pathways, because of the existing pressure gradients the saturation changes accordingly. In the lungs, where the capillary blood contacts the alveolar air, the oxygen saturation is maximal and in the blood leaving the tissues where oxygen is used it is minimal. Actual values depend mainly on the specific relationships between pO_2 and haemoglobin saturation known as oxygen-haemoglobin dissociation curve, but also on the pH, temperature and pCO_2 in blood.

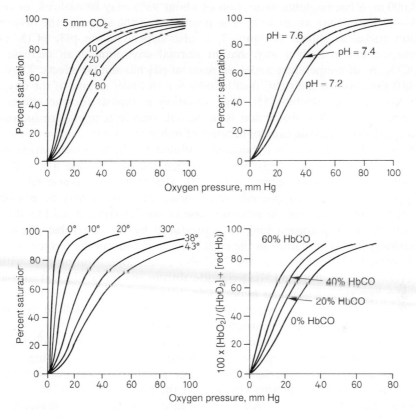

Fig. 3. Effects of partial pressure of carbon dioxide (pCO$_2$), blood acidity (pII), temperature and carboxyhaemoglobin (HbCO) concentration on the oxygen-haemoglobin dissociation curve [From ref. 55, p. 159].

The oxygen-haemoglobin dissociation curve (fig. 3) has a sigmoidal shape, with a steep initial slope, corresponding to low pO$_2$ values and a flat portion, corresponding to the high end of the pO$_2$ values. This shape of the curve has considerable physiological significance. Over the flat portion of the curve, corresponding to the pO$_2$ in lungs at sea level, even considerable fluctuations in pAO$_2$, depending on breathing pattern or other reasons, do not interfere with the haemoglobin saturation or the oxygen content of arterial blood. Over the steep portion of the curve, corresponding to the pO$_2$ at the tissue level of circulation, even minimal changes in oxygen tension allow for considerable unloading of oxygen for diffusion into the cells. It may be seen that due to the sigmoidal shape of the dissociation curve even at a pAO$_2$ of 75 mm Hg, corresponding to an altitude of

2,000 m, a haemoglobin saturation of about 93% may be realized, or only 3–4% lower than at sea level. The position and the shape of the dissociation curve, as shown in figure 3, is also dependent on pH, pCO_2 and temperature in such a way that in normal environment an increase of pCO_2, or of temperature and a decrease of pH has similar effects. They all shift the curve to the right, thus helping for an easier release of the oxygen bound to haemoglobin [55]. This situation is typical for the effects of exercise when CO_2 production is increased, muscle temperature increases and pH may decrease rapidly because of enhanced lactate release in blood. At altitude, however, the hypocapnia induced by the hyperventilation may in fact have adverse effects on the oxygen release, because a low pCO_2 shifts the dissociation curve to the left. However, the adverse effects of hypocapnia on the oxygen release at moderate altitude may be compensated by an increase of the concentration of the 2,3-DPG in red blood cells with the acclimatization [56]. It is produced by the anaerobic glycolytic pathway and is contained in the erythrocytes, favouring the oxygen release in hypocapnic background. The 2,3-DPG blood concentration rises within several days at altitude [57]. Evidently during the initial days at altitude, when hyperventilation and hypocapnia do exist, but the 2,3-DPG level is still relatively low, the oxygen release at the tissue level will be impaired even if enough oxygen is carried in the blood.

The haemoglobin concentration and red cell count in blood during the first days at altitude progressively increase. At the very beginning of the acclimatization this is a relative and not an absolute rise, because it is more due to a decrease of plasma volume, i.e. the haemoconcentration, then to a new red cell production. Although erythropoetic activity increases in the early hours of the acclimatization to hypoxia [58], the maximum rate is achieved after 1 or 2 weeks and red cell mass may still increase after 1 year of residence at altitude. Hence, the increased haemoglobin concentration and red cell count, while very important parameters of acclimatization, belong to the slower mechanisms of adaptation to hypoxia.

Obviously, the increased red cell mass is basically an adaptive mechanism, increasing the oxygen transport capacity of the arterial blood. The erythrocytes are not only carriers of haemoglobin, but they also determine the dimension of the respiratory contact area for loading or unloading of oxygen in blood. A potential adverse effect, however, of the increased red cell mass is the rise of the blood viscosity, which in turn may lead to a considerable elevation of the flow resistance in the blood pathways, over some critical haematocrit value. Once again a biological compromise is needed for optimal adaptation during acclimatization between the oxygen-carrying capacity of the blood and the flow resistance in the blood pathways.

The degree of the polycythaemic response is related to the level of altitude. Up to an elevation of 3,660 m the haemoglobin level increases in a linear relation to altitude [8]. In our experience with athletes, trained for 2 or 3 weeks at altitudes between 1,800 and 2,600 m, the increase of red cell count and haemoglobin concentration was in the range of 10–15% [59, 60]. Similar data were published by Roskamm et al. [29]. After 4 weeks in Mexico City the Hb concentration in two groups of German athletes increased on average by about 15%, the red cell count by 8.5%, and the haematocrit by 8%. In a group of athletes, training at 3,350 m during 3 weeks, an increase of haemoglobin to 18.6 g/dl, or about 24% over the normal values was reported by Zima et al. [61]. It is of note that absolute peak values were found not at altitude, but several days after coming down, at normal environment. Three weeks later the haemoglobin concentration remained still considerably higher than normal at 16.7 g/dl.

A very important feature of the adaptation to exercise at altitude in the context of sports training and performances is that most of the physiological mechanisms involved in the struggle for oxygen also need oxygen, thus contributing indirectly for an enhanced energy cost of exercise. Some of them have controversial effects at different sites of the oxygen transport chain or some critical levels, after which adverse physiological effects may appear. As a typical example we may take the hyperventilation response during exercise at altitude. At an altitude of 2,000 m the partial pressure of oxygen in the alveolar air is decreased to 75 mm Hg, or about 25% below the sea level value. To compensate a proportional increase of the lung ventilation is needed, at rest and during exercise as well. At rest the additional energy cost of breathing will be negligibly small, because the 'oxygen price' of lung function at rest is estimated to be as low as 1 ml oxygen per liter of ventilation. So 2 or 3 liters additional ventilation will not be any burden for the oxygen balance of organism. During exercise, however, the situation may be very much different, because, depending on the intensity of exercise the ventilation may be tremendously increased and the 'O_2 price' per liter of air ventilated rises exponentially with the ventialtion rate. If contemporary training is considered with a typical intensity, in most cases around the anaerobic threshold (at heart rates in the range of 170–180 beats/min), a ventilation in the range of 130–150 litres/min is to be expected even at sea level. At an altitude of 2,000 m 25% more, or 32–38 litres/min of air will be needed to compensate for the lower pAO_2 in lungs According to Shephard [13], the 'oxygen cost' of this additional ventilation will be as high as 7 ml per litre/min, or about 250 ml O_2/min, which is significant. In fact, the cost might be even higher, because hyperventilation in a hypocapnic environment may provoke bronchospasm thus increasing the resistance of the airways in the lung. According to

Newhouse [62] at a pCO_2 of 25 mm Hg the energy cost of hyperventilation was 68% higher than in normocapnia (pCO_2 45 mm Hg). Evidently, the additional cost of breathing at altitude may be accepted as a 'reasonable price' only if the additional oxygen flux to the working muscles, due to the added respiratory effort, is greater than the increase of oxygen consumption in the respiratory muscles. Furthermore, it is quite clear that at workloads approaching the maximal aerobic power ($\dot{V}O_2$ max) if an additional oxygen price is to be paid for the respiratory work the only possibility to keep on breathing is to limit accordingly the oxygen flux to the muscles engaged in external work, i.e. in exercise. The net result under the circumstances has to be a lower performance at altitude in sport events depending on the aerobic power. In events depending relatively more on anaerobic power, like sprint running, long or triple jumps, cycling, short distance skating, etc., the handicap of hypoxia may be largely compensated by the lower air density and hence lower aerodynamic resistance at altitude. In these kinds of sports, the moderate altitude can have a favourable effect on the athletic performance.

During prolonged acclimatization and training at altitude there is a tendency to normalize the cardiorespiratory functions at rest and during submaximal exercise as well, but the maximum aerobic power ($\dot{V}O_2$ max) of trained athletes, according to different research groups: (1) may not change significantly [21, 37, 40, 48, 63]; (2) while increasing does not attain sea level values [20, 24, 26, 29, 49, 64]; and (3) may recover to sea level or even slightly better values [14, 65].

In our experience with international level athletes of different sports (altogether 118 subjects, preparing for the Olympic games in Mexico City) $\dot{V}O_2$ max at altitude tended to return to its prealtitude level after 4–6 weeks of training at 2,000 m [66]. The ergometric performance, however, remained on average 2–4% lower than in Sofia (550 m above sea level).

The physiological background for a nearly perfect compensation of the impairments towards the oxygen transport at altitude after 4–6 weeks of acclimatization are presented by the increased oxygen capacity of blood and the particular shape of the dissociation curve shifted to the right, as described above, by the specific training effect of the hyperventilation during exercise on the respiratory system [67–72], by the adaptive changes of the regional blood flow in lungs and in muscles, by the increased myoglobin concentration in muscles [8, 73], and by the enhanced oxidative capacity of muscles due to raised enzyme activity in mitochondria [73, 74]. With the acclimatization the hypocapnia is gradually diminished due to the trend to normalization of the lung ventilation at rest and during submaximal exercise. The initial blood alkalosis is eliminated by enhanced excretion of plasma bicarbonate through the kidney [29]. Thus, the acid-base balance is restored, although at the expense of a lowered buffering capacity of the blood. The lactate concentration in blood during submaximal exercise, which at acute exposure to hypoxia is higher than at sea level [63, 75, 76], tends to decrease with acclimatization to altitude, due to a lower rate of net lactate release at comparable workloads [77].

The elevated energy cost of the oxygen transport at altitude, however, particularly at near maximal training intensities and during competition, remains a considerable handicap for the athletic performance at altitude. Its relative importance is proportional to the duration of the respective activity. This can be demonstrated using performance times from the Olympic games in Mexico City, 1968.

The running times in the sprint events were equal or better than the world records of that time. Some of them are still, after 22 years of intensive development of the athletics worldwide, unbeaten (43.86 on 400 m, 2.56.16 on relay race 4 × 400 m, 8.90 long jump[1]). Others are until now among the 6 best performances of all times in the track and field rankings (9.95 on 100 m, 19.83 and 19.92 on 200 m, 43.97, second best time on 400 m, 38.39 on relay race 4 × 100 m). In the 800 m race, the Olympic performance was equal to the world record at that time, but was not as outstandingly high as the above-cited result in the 400 m and shorter events. It may be speculated that on distances shorter than 800 m the relatively small hypoxic handicap is largely outbalanced by the lower air resistance, thus allowing for excellent performances. The 800 m distance, or the time of about 100 s, appears to be a borderline after which the hypoxia is more critical than the lower air resistance at altitude. The performances on distances longer than 800 m were definitely worse than world records. The difference was as small as 1.8 s (0.85%) in the 1,500 m, but as great as 650 s (8.35%) in the marathon race. The above results are of interest not only as a practical confirmation of scientific considerations, but also as a base for optimal planning of training at altitude.

The comparison of swimming times confirmed the above conclusions. The 100 m time was slightly faster than the world record, but the 1,500 m performance was definitely worse.

Is There Any Reason for Training at Altitude?

In our opinion there are at least two reasons to answer 'Yes':
(1) The environment at altitude 2,000–3,000 m may be very favourable for training in sports based on speed and power.

---

[1] The world record in long jump set in Mexico 1968 was recently broken by Mike Powell, in Tokyo, summer 1991.

(2) The adaptive changes during training at altitude may prove useful for the endurance capacity in a normal, sea level, environment.

The favourable environmental conditions for sprint training at altitude do not need extended discussion. Inasmuch as speed and power performances depend almost exclusively on anaerobic energy metabolism there is no reason to expect physiological limitations due to hypoxia if training methods are properly adjusted to allow longer recovery time within a training session and in general. Further, the physical and biomechanical advantages, created by the lower air resistance and force of gravity at altitude, although small, contribute to enhanced performances, as demonstrated by the sprint and jump events in Mexico City, 1968. Recently, Karvonen and co-workers presented experimental data confirming the positive effects of altitude training on speed- and speed-endurance performances of sprinters and on the anaerobic power and capacity [78–81]. They conclude that altitude training is equivalent to supramaximal training loads used for developing the neuromuscular system and anaerobic energy processes required for speed production. In a sea-level environment, supramaximal sprints or long jumps are pratically impossible, unless incidentally, with a strong fair wind. The only other possibility is running on negative slopes, but there are biomechanical considerations against this, not to mention a more prosaic reason that all normal athletic tracks are strictly horizontal. If a negative slope is needed it must be found out of the stadium, on normal roads, or parks, and therefore may not provide an optimal running surface. At altitude the sprinter may run faster on a normal running track, preserving the conventional biomechanical structure of the specific motor activity (distance running or accelerating for jumping), hardly possible on a negative slope track.

If we now return to the adaptive changes during training at altitude, as a base for enhanced endurance capacity in normal environment, it appears that some adaptations are likely to be very useful indeed. For example, the enhanced oxygen capacity of blood, due to the increased Hb concentration and red cell count, should enhance oxygen transport because Hb saturation will be maximal at normal pAO_2. The ventilation of the alveolar space will be accomplished with lower breathing frequency and/or tidal volume, as compared to respiration at altitude at any given level of exercise intensity. Hence, the energy cost of breathing will be lower and relatively more oxygen may be used for external work. Simultaneously, the CO_2 elimination will be normalized. Thus, the adverse effects of hypocapnia on the tissue oxygenation and on the regulation of ventilation will be removed automatically. As a result, a better endurance performance might be expected after acclimatization and training at altitude. However, while the above physiological facts are generally well established, there is no unequivocal answer on the question how maximum endurance performance at sea level is affected following altitude training. The general consensus is that considerable individual differences do exist in the adaptability of athletes to altitude. Some of the top athletes might be more vulnerably affected by altitude than others who are less conditioned [82], though there are contradictory opinions as well [11].

The Controversies

Some investigators who have studied top-level athletes feel that if a highly trained athlete is close to his individual maximum of trainability, altitude training might not further increase an already high capacity [26, 83]. Moreover, it might be dangerous to try it. On the other hand, others believe that altitude training is a powerful method for improving the oxygen transport and the endurance capacity, expecially useful for highly trained athletes who have come very close to the limits of their training programs in normal conditions [11]. For them, altitude training may provide a way to enhance the physiological effect of exercise without further increasing the already very high volume of training loads on the musculoskeletal system.

The controversies on this subject appeared from the very beginning of the intensive research on altitude training before the Olympic Games in Mexico and now, 25 years later, they continue to be unresolved.

Balke et al. [82] suggested that following altitude training, 'the top athlete's physiologic capacity will be boosted and he should be able to utilize this advantage if called upon by adequate muscle action. Here, apparently, are the limitations: during the period of time in which physiological compensation for the reduced atmospheric oxygen tension might gradually become more adequate, the power output of the muscles trained for maximum effort is definitely diminished because of the reduced oxygen supply. This period, then, is practically comparable with a period of muscular detraining...' Despite greater general strain, the local demands may actually be inadequate for an optimal muscle training.

Jensen and Fisher [84], after a short review on altitude training, concluded that: 'there seems to be no evidence that perforamnce is improved by training at a higher altitude for a performance at a lower altitude, with the possible exception that the anaerobic processes of the body may be improved slightly by the high altitude training. Athletes who train at high altitude do not perform better at sea level.'

A similar position was defended by Saltin [85] in 1986. He concluded, after presenting recent experimental data, that: 'all these data do not speak

in favour of any special positive effects of training at altitude for aerobic
performance, as rather on the contrary. It may in fact be difficult for a top
trained endurance athlete to maintain his/her fitness during a more prolonged stay at altitude although the training is kept at the highest possible
level. In less than optimally trained subjects training at altitude may result
in improvements. The question is, however, whether the same increases
may not have been achieved by training at sea level?'

Jackson and Sharkey [86] concluded their review on altitude training
and human performance in a similar way: 'Altitude training is known to
affect events that are aerobic and it still does not appear to be advantageous for the sea level athlete to condition at altitude.'

In contrast, in 1988, Nowacki [12] presented very positive results from
altitude training of the German national rowing team at Silvretta See,
2,040 m above sea level. He firmly believed that altitude training has great
potential to improve endurance performance of Olympic level athletes. For
this reason, he suggested that altitude training has to be considered as a
violation of the fair play rules and concluded that appropriate limitations
have to be inserted in the Olympic Charter and in the World championships regulations to prevent altitude training before championships 'for
otherwise the rich sport nations will have an additional advantage.'

Lychatz [11] in a review on the development of training methods in
endurance sports during the Olympic cycle 1985–1988 accepted as a
starting point of his presentation on the hypoxia training the following
thesis: 'In endurance sports the hypoxia training is a key factor which may
not be neglected. Otherwise, the world poll position will be lost.'

According to Suslov [87] the most probable reason for the polarization
of the existing opinions on altitude training among physiologists and in
practical experience of trainers as well, may be the shortage of well-
established methods for endurance training at altitude to cope with the
complexity of adaptation of athletes to the combined stress of hypoxia and
vigorous exercise.

The fact itself that many controversial results were found suggests that
factors other than altitude are contributing to the end-result, which is
evaluated through physiological parameters or sport performances. All
those factors, generally known, measurable and routinely used as descrip-
tors of training loads like volume, intensity or structure of training may
have different relative importance at different altitudes at different times
during acclimatization and according to the individual pattern of adaptation to altitude. Because of the complexity of the mechanisms of physiological adaptation it may be rather difficult to optimise the process of training
at altitude in general and in every individual case as well. With this in
mind, it is not difficult to imagine that quite often the end-result of altitude

training may depend not only on altitude itself, but also on the complex interrelationships between altitude and the imposed training loads. It may be positive only if the cumulative stress is well within the limits of the adaptive capacity of organism. If not, negative effects are not to be excluded.

The Bulgarian Experience

In Bulgaria, research on altitude training started as early as 1952 and in our first publications [59, 60] we recommended training at moderate altitudes for increasing oxygen transport and endurance capacity. Since 1967, when the Altitude Training Centre at Belmeken, in Rila mountain, 2,050 m above sea level was built, thousands of athletes have trained there. Mostly, altitude training was carried out during the periods for general preparation using predominantly nonspecific exercises like field running or skiing in the winter, climbing steep slopes, free swimming, power and power-endurance exercises, stationary rowing, etc. Some athletes (wrestlers, boxers, rowers, canoeists, biathlonists, orienteerers) also used the facilities for specific training several weeks before important competitions like the Olympic Games or World championships. In the period 1967–1968 all Olympic teams preparing for Mexico trained at Belmeken. At that time extensive follow-up studies were made on athletes of different sports during acclimatization at Belmeken and on some athletes in Mexico as well.

Generally, we have found that after a week of acclimatization almost normal training was possible, despite the existing limitations imposed by the decreased aerobic power and the higher energy cost of exercise if individualised training loads rather than team work sessions were considered. Allowing for more freedom of the individual training loads to cope with the general scheme of training and using slightly longer recovery times, combined or not with shorter work intervals, the coaches managed to avoid overstrain or health problems during acclimatization. In the initial phases of the altitude training some athletes had problems establishing a convenient breathing pattern in step with the specific motor activity pace.

After 2 weeks at altitude, the athletes trained according to their normal training schedules, except that 'the cruising speed' in longer duration exercises was slightly lower than in a normal environment, the greater the duration the greater the difference.

The observed changes in exercise capacity after the first 2–3 days at altitude, compared to Sofia (550 m above sea level), were in most cases minimal, i.e. $\dot{V}o_2$ max decreased by about 2–4%, maximal ergometric performance (bicycle ergometer) decreased by about 2–6%. Some athletes from the wrestling and boxing teams did not show any decrease in either of these tests. It is of note, however, that most of the athletes had previously trained at altitudes of 1,600–1,800 m and were more or less accustomed to exercise at altitude.

After 4–6 weeks of altitude training $\dot{V}O_2$ max and ergometric performance tended to reach or slightly exceed the prealtitude values observed in Sofia. However, some athletes, even after 6 weeks, still remained at a 1–3% inferior level.

It was concluded that an altitude of about 2,000 m does not impose severe impairments on training or athletic performance but nevertheless slightly inferior performances should be expected in the endurance events in the Mexico Olympic Games. As discussed above, this is exactly what occurred.

At that time we did not assess the physiological parameters or athletic performances during reacclimatization after altitude training, because our interest was the performance in Mexico. However, during the more than 20 years since the Mexico Olympics, we have routinely tested international level athletes before and after training camps at Belmeken (2,050 m). On average, a slight but consistent positive effect on the aerobic power and on the maximal ergometric work capacity was found. Unfortunately, these were not strictly controlled experiments. Therefore, the results are not conclusive. In most cases it is impossible to distinguish between the cumulative effects of altitude and the training itself. For this reason, we shall present here only some data from a follow-up study of the national rowing team over a 15-month period during their preparation for the Olympic Games in Los Angeles, where training and altitude effects might be separated.

The study was conducted from November 1982 to February 1984. During this time, 32 rowers were tested at 2- to 3-month intervals, using a standard progressive test protocol on the bicycle ergometer until exhaustion, for determination of $\dot{V}O_2$ max and other physiological parameters.

Over the above period the athletes trained together in common training camps. Only in January 1983 were they divided into two groups: one consisting of 20 rowers, who trained for 3 weeks at an altitude of 2,050 m (Belmeken group) and the second comprising 12 rowers who trained during the same 3 weeks at sea level on the Black sea shore (Sozopol group). The training programs of both groups were identical and were aimed at general conditioning, using mainly strength- and power-endurance exercises and field running, usual for that period of the annual training program of the team. Immediately after the training camps both groups returned to Sofia (550 m above sea level) and were tested over 2 consecutive days.

For the rest of the year both groups trained together, mostly at sea

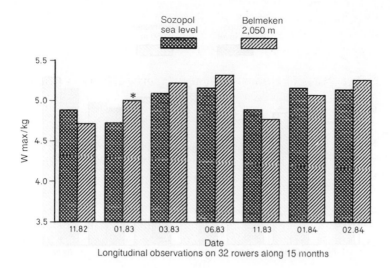

Fig. 4. Maximum ergometric performance (W max/kg) after training at altitude or at
sea level. Explanations in text.

level, or in places not higher than 500–600 m and were routinely tested
several times. In January 1984, both groups trained for 3 weeks at
Belmeken (at 2,050 m) and were tested twice after returning to Sofia: once
during the first 3 days after coming down (Test Jan. 1984) and again 2
weeks later (Test Feb. 1984).

Averaged test data are presented in figures 4–6. Statistically significant
differences between groups are marked by an asterisk.

The main results may be summarized as follows:

(1) After 3 weeks of training at altitude, in January 1983, the aerobic
power of the Belmeken group was increased, despite the prevailing anaerobic rather than aerobic character of exercises during the trianing camp.
Ergometric performance was also improved, despite lower anaerobic capacity (lower maximal lactate values) after returning from Belmeken.

The aerobic power of the Sozopol group, coming from sea level, was
not increased. In fact, it was slightly decreased, as expected, since the
majority of training efforts during this early period of the annual program
were concentrated on power rather than on endurance, as mentioned
above. The ergometric performance and the maximum lactate level were
unchanged.

(2) Surprisingly, the differences between the two groups seemed to
remain for months after returning to joint training. It is unlikely that these
differences are due to a direct residual effect of the relatively very short time

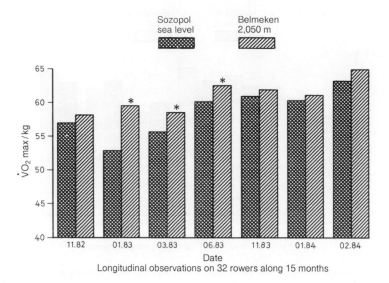

Fig. 5. Maximum oxygen uptake ($\dot{V}O_2$ max/kg) after training at altitude or at sea level. Explanations in text.

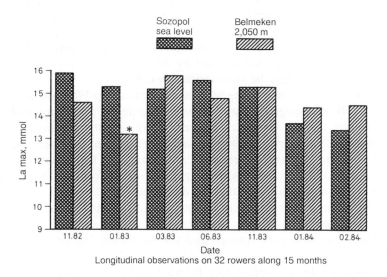

Fig. 6. Maximum blood lactate concentration after training at altitude or at sea level. Explanations in text.

of the respective training camps at altitude and at sea level. It is well known that after returning to normal conditions most of the adaptive changes to the altitude disappear at a rate similar to that of the gain, i.e. within days or weeks. Therefore, the superior position of the Belmeken group for the next several months, as compared to the Sozopol group, may have been due to the better quality of training, as a result of their enhanced aerobic power.

(3) When both groups went together to altitude in January 1984, the test results of both were similar to the 1983 postaltitude data of the Belmeken group. It is noteworthy that the highest values of $\dot{V}O_2$ max were observed not immediately after coming down, but after 2 weeks of training in Sofia. During this time the maximal blood lactate concentration remained unchanged on a slightly lower level than prealtitude.

In our experience, the above results are typical when favourable conditions for training and living at altitude exist. They are not, however, automatically guaranteed simply by taking a team to altitude. Negative results are not excluded. Although there can be many reasons for a failure of altitude training, typically an underestimation of the training loads occurs during the most vulnerable initial period of acclimatization, when self-control may be disturbed and training may easily be overdosed.

Some Physiological Reasons for the Difficult
Management of Training at Altitude

The main physiological reason for the difficult management of training at altitude is the well-known fact that top athletes train mostly in a very narrow space of adaptability, where the borderline between under- and overloading is most delicate. The environmental factors are always contributing to the training loads. Though usually neglected, they actually are intrinsic ingredients of the total physiological strain during exercise. At altitude the lower air density and the hypoxia, though both depending on a common physical factor (the barometric pressure), have separate effects on the motor activity and on the physiological strain during training. As mentioned above, the athlete may run faster short distances, or jump further at altitude, but the recovery time after strenuous exercises will be slightly longer and the cruising speed for long distances will be inevitably slower due to hypoxia. The problem is how to design a creative training program at altitude, if the muscles may rest underloaded, due to the limitations of the oxygen supply?

It is evident that the spontaneous correction of the rate of activity (slower pace or shorter stride in running, diminished power of strokes in rowing and swimming, etc.) according to the perceived exertion will not do. An inappropriate correction, because of an overestimation of the real physiological strain, will lead to a lower training efficiency. But even an appropriate pace control, based on the overall strain during exercise, may not be enough for an optimal stress on the motor system at altitude because the oxygen supply is the rate-limiting factor not the muscle itself.

An important point for understanding the problems of altitude training is the informational aspect of the adaptation to exercise in a hypoxic environment. It is well known that the adaptation of the organism to a very large range of environmental conditions is possible due to the sophisticated network of physiological sensors permanently receiving and transferring to the central nervous system (CNS) specific information on the environment and on the organism itself, thus allowing for adaptive behaviour and respective changes of physiological parameters at the local level, or in the whole organism.

During exercise, the main input channels are those supplying information on the parameters of the motor activity, on the functions of respiration and circulation and on the changes of the physicochemical properties of the body fluids and the blood. Generally, while at steady state, there are well-established correlation and synchronization of the informational flux through the different channels, allowing for a rapid processing of information in the CNS, for making decisions and for sending back appropriate driving impulses to the motor and to the vegetative systems.

At altitude during the initial phases of acclimatization, and at sea level during reacclimatization after returning from altitude, several days are needed for adjustment (respectively, for readjustment) and for fine tuning of the informational network to cope with the disturbed proportionality of the signals coming from the motor system (work rate, speed of movement, strength of muscle contractions, metabolic rate), from the cardiorespiratory system (respiration rate, heart rate, blood pressure), from the blood (pCO_2, pH, pO_2), and others.

The motor system is a dominant source of information during exercise. Therefore, the real physiological strain due to exercise at altitude may be easily underestimated if the motor system is not habitually stressed, according to sea level standards, despite the maximal exertion of the vegetative systems. As a consequence the athlete may be forced beyond his habitual limits of exhaustion, to acute overstrain or to overtraining. A dramatic illustration of the situation, which is seldom, if ever seen elsewhere, were world class athletes collapsing at the finals of middle and long distance races in the Mexico Olympics and recovering under oxygen administration.

During reacclimatization after altitude training a similar, while not so dramatic situation due to informational disorders does exist during the first days of functional readjustments of the organism. Then it may be difficult, even for top athletes, to set an optimal pace of exercise and to reestablish the habitual breathing pattern in step with motor activity due to the adopted (corrected for altitude environment) 'new scale of estimation' of the severity of physical exertion.

Training Guidelines

The consequences of the altitude environment for sport training may be summarized as follows:

(1) Altitude does not interfere with short-term exercises, depending mianly on anaerobic energy supply. The motor system may be optimally stressed during activities shorter than 100 s.

(2) The racing speed in track and field and swimming events longer than 100 s, depending predominantly on aerobic power and endurance, may be 1–8% slower than that at sea level. The longer the distance, the greater the difference. The motor system may not be stressed optimally, because work rate is limited by the reduced oxygen supply and the resulting general strain rather than by the muscle power or muscle oxidative capacity.

The same is not true for cycling or ice skating, as the hypoxic handicap is largely compensated by the lower air resistance at the respective racing speeds in these sports.

(3) Recovery time after intensive training loads may be slightly longer at altitude.

(4) The most vulnerable period during a training camp at altitude is likely to be the initial phase of acclimatization, when self-control, based on feedback information, may be disturbed and the physiological strain of training may be underestimated.

(5) After returning from altitude several days are also needed for reacclimatization and readjustment of the feedback mechanisms accordingly for an optimal level of control and coordination of motor action and vegetative functions.

Based on the above considerations the following guidelines may be useful in altitude training for performance in normal environment:

(1) Speed and power training may not create any particular problems. Training schedules may be almost identical with sea level programs; however, slightly longer recovery intervals are recommended. When work intervals are longer than 1 min, the number of repetitions should be reduced as well, but speed should be held at the highest possible level for the training distance. Otherwise, the bonuses of the lower air resistance for specific speed development will not be used optimally.

(2) The optimization of endurance training is more complicated because the habitual pace of running is impossible due to hypoxia. Long distances may be run with a speed 0.3–0.4 m/sec slower than at sea level [10]. The expected handicap may be more than 2 min over 10 km, about 50 s over 5 km, 10–15 s over 2 km and 4–8 s over 1 km, despite maximal efforts. The problem is how to prevent the adverse effects of the lower speed of running on the motor system, which in fact is not stressed to its capacity. The only possibility, in my opinion, is to avoid as much as possible training on the competition distance, running instead fractions of it at an equal or slightly faster pace than when running the whole distance at sea level. Thus, the working muscles will be stressed to their capacity in step with the effective maximal (or optimal) strain of the oxygen transport typical for the altitude and needed for improving endurance training. Evidently, the structure of training has to be at intervals or intermittent. The relationships between work and rest, or between fast and slow running intervals, have to be arranged on an individual basis according to the annual training program and for the particular period or microcycle. Generally, the work bouts have to be relatively shorter in the earlier phases of the acclimatization, the number of repetitions diminished, and the recovery time prolonged. In other words, the total volume of the work will be reduced, the mean intensity (total work/total time of a training session) will be lower, but the intensity of the work intervals will be slightly higher than during tempo runs over the respective whole distance at sea level. During the stay at altitude, the total work volume and the mean intensity of training will be increased gradually at the expense of the recovery intervals, aiming towards a structure of training similar to sea level.

The duration of the work intervals for an individual athlete is a matter of experience and empirical adjustment to the individual's adaptability. As a rule, a marathon runner should be able to run at altitude for 12–15 km at the sea-level pace for the marathon distance and a 10,000 m runner for 3–5 km at a speed comparable to the sea-level pace. The above recommendations are based on a mathematical analysis of the relationships speed:distance using Olympic records in track and field for distances between 400 m and marathon from Mexico 1968. The rationale is the well-known negative correlation between distance and speed of running, which in the range from 400 m to marathon may be well approximated by relatively simple biexponential functions:

$$Y = A1 \cdot \exp(B1 \cdot X) + A2 \cdot \exp(B2 \cdot X), \tag{1}$$

where $Y = \text{Ln [distance (m)]}$; $X = $ running speed (m/s), and
A1, B1, A2, B2 = empirical constants, or:

$$Y = C1 \cdot \exp(D1 \cdot X) + C2 \cdot \exp(D2 \cdot X), \tag{2}$$

where Y = running speed (m/s); X = Ln [distance (m)], and $C1, D1, C2, D2$ = empirical constants.

Using the Olympic records from Mexico City, 1968 and a standard iterative computational program for PC HP9816, we calculated the following values for the empirical constants of the above equations:

(1)		(2)	
$A1 = 95.006$	$B1 = -0.61343$	$C1 = 756.698$	$D1 = -0.97664$
$A2 = 7.108$	$B2 = -0.02544$	$C2 = 10.603$	$D2 = -0.07081$

The graphs of the above equations (fig. 7, 8), may serve as nomograms for a rapid orientation concerning the respective interrelationships. For a more precise estimation, the respective equations have to be used. With them it is an easy problem to estimate the approximate distance which may be run by a top-level athlete at an altitude of 2,250 m at any given speed in the range from 5 to 9 m/s, or inversely: which speed may be run by the same athlete for any appropriate distance in the range from 400 m to marathon. The 'appropriate' distance is of course a distance in the range of those, habitually run in training at sea level, according to the specialization of the respective athlete. Evidently, the same reasoning is true for the application of both equations. For example, if the winner of the marathon in Mexico 1968 would have liked to run there with sea level speed for marathon (5.43 m/s, for that time) he should not be able to run more than 14–15 km at this pace. Or, inversely, if he wanted to run 15 km, the appropriate speed for this distance at that altitude should be about 5.4 m/s.

If the sea level performance of an athlete is not exactly comparable with the world best performances, evidently a correction will be needed for a more realistic recommendation. The correction factor may be easily calculated, dividing the individual's best performance by the world record for the respective distance. For example, if the marathon runner wanted to run at altitude a distance of 10 km with an adequate training speed, he might calculate, using the appropriate equation, a recommended speed of 5.62 m/s. But if his personal best time for this distance was not close to 27.39.4 or 6.03 m/s (the world record at that time), but only 30 min or 5.56 m/s, the correction factor $= 5.56/6.03 = 0.92$ has to be applied to the calculated 5.62 m/s to receive the final result: $5.62 \cdot 0.92 = 5.17$ m/s, or

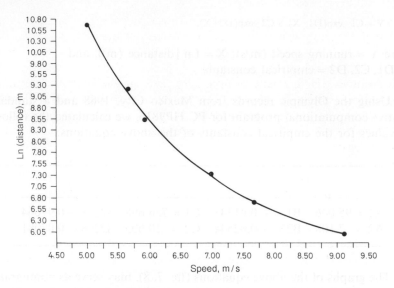

Fig. 7. Graphic presentation of the relationships between running speed and Ln of distance at 2,250 m above sea level. (Database: Olympic Games winners results, Mexico, 1968.) Explanations in text.

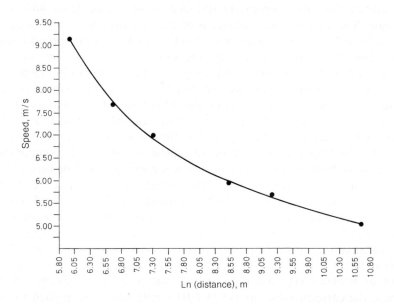

Fig. 8. Graphic presentation of the inverse function as in figure 7. Explanations in text.

3 min 13 s per km. Evidently, analogous considerations have to be applied, when searching for the optimal distance to be run at a given speed.

Of course, the above equations are only valid for altitudes close to those of Mexico City. Unfortunately, there are no comparable data for other altitudes, but it might be estimated than an additional handicap of 1% should be used for every 100 m additional altitude up to 3,000–3,200 m. In the above example, if the training camp was not in Mexico City but 400 m higher, in Tolouca, the calculated training pace of 5.17 m/s should have to be diminished by an addiitonal 4%, or 0.21 m/s. So the recommended pace will be: 5.17–0.21 = 4.96 m/s or 3 min 22 s per km.

As shown above, the possible speed of running is progressively diminshed with altitude, so that altitudes much higher than 2,300 m are not feasible for training to improve performance at a sea-level environment.

The above recommendations, based on mathematical analysis, may also be applied to submaxial running paces, expressed as a percent of maximum. Evidently, at altitude the sea level maximum would not be a valid base for calculations, but determining a new, altitude base, through conventional testing in the early acclimatization period may not be optimal either. Using a sea-level database and the above equations, it may be possible to plan training loads more precisely optimally applying sea-level experience in the new environment. The general outline of the training program thus created must be further individualized, according to the actual adaptability of athletes during the acclimatization at altitude using appropriate information concerning functional state, performance capacity, health and total well-being of the subjects. Perferably objective, rather than subjective, data should be used, because, as mentioned above, the self-estimation in the initial period of acclimatization may not be reliable enough, even in subjects with some previous experience with altitude training. A reliable source of information could be the heart rate total for a known, measurable training load, if recorded precisely during the respective activity with an appropriate testing device.

As a general rule for the training program at altitude caution is recommended by most investigators for the first several days at altitude [10, 30, 32, 88], but there are different opinions as well [82, 89]. In my opinion, it is best not to force the events during the initial adaptation at altitude, allowing for a slower but safer build up of the performance capacity in the new environment. After the first week an incremental approach is recommended toward the habitual training loads at sea level, so that during the third week a normal training program could be realized with only the necessary adaptation of the running speed (or, more gener ally, of the training intensity) to the restrictions imposed by the hypoxia, as discussed above.

It is generally accepted that repeated altitude training helps to accelerate the adaptive processes at altitude and for the cumulative effect of the altitude on the organism. For this reason, it is recommended to organize more than one altitude camp during a training year, preferably three, the last one just before the most important competition [11]. The minimal duration of an altitude training camp for endurance sports is recommended to be 3 weeks [88]. Based on our experience, this seems to be optimal. Longer camps may create problems, due not to hypoxia, but to other factors (including climatological, meteorological, psychological, sociological) interfering with training, not to mention training facilities, which may not be optimal for specific sports, even in places with very good general equipment.

During reacclimatization from altitude training, the performance capacity of athletes is generally improved, but there are some fluctuations around the typical trend which may lead to unexpected and sometimes disappointing results. According to Bishon [88], there are three favourable periods for sport performances after altitude training:

(1) During the first 3–10 h immediately after returning.

(2) During the 4th to 5th day (in most cases).

(3) Between 12 and 30 days after returning from altitude.

In contrast, Poehlitz [10] does not recommend any attempt for maximal performances during the first 5 days after coming down. The best performance in middle distance events, in his opinion, may be recorded 24–28 days after returning to a normal environment. The positive effects of altitude training may remain for 6 or more weeks if athletes are properly trained, with intensive training loads during this time.

In our experience, the best results immediately after returning from altitude are possible in speed and power exercises (sprinting, jumping, throwing), but probably not in endurance events where athletes have problems in reestablishing the optimal working pace at sea level environment after adopting a slower pace at altitude. The most unfavourable period for competitions seems to be the time between the 3rd and 5th days. After that, the performance gradually improves peaking at about the 4th week after coming down. A relatively high performance level may be preserved for 6 or more weeks if training intensity is kept at a demanding level.

Conclusion

Despite considerable controversy both in scientific publications and in practical experience, the potential of altitude training remains an attractive possibility to enhance the performance capacity at sea level. It is a challenge for both researchers and coaches to establish reliable methods to optimize training at altitude in order to minimize the intrinsic incompatibility of hypoxia and aerobic performance.

References

1   Proceedings of the Alma-Ata Symposium: Acclimatization and training of athletes at altitude (in Russian). Alma-Ata, 1965.
2   Margaria R (ed): International Symposium: Exercise at altitude, Milan 1966. Milan, Excerpta Medica Foundation, 1967.
3   Goddart RF (ed): International Symposium: The effects of Altitude on Physical Performance, Albuquerque, 1966. Chicago, Athletic Institute, 1967.
4   Schoenhoelzer G (ed): International Symposium: Sports in Medium Altitude, Magglingen, 1966. Schweiz Z Sportmed 1966;14.
5   Zimkin NW, Farfel WS (eds): Proceedings of 9th Allunion Conference on Physiology, Morphology, Biochemistry and Biomechanic of Muscle Activity, vol IV. Problems of Acclimatization (in Russian). Moscow, 1966. (Russ).
6   Proceedings of the International Symposium of the Socialist Countries: Problems of Sport Training (in Russian). Moscow, 1967.
7   Craig AB: Olympics 1968. A post mortem. Med Sci Sports 1969;I:177–183.
8   Heath D, Williams DR: Man at High Altitude: The Pathophysiology of Acclimatization and Adaptation. Edinburgh, Churchill Livingstone, 1981, pp 287–288.
9   Banister R: Chairmans opening remarks. Br J Sports Med 1974;8:3–4.
10   Poehlitz L: Praktische Erfahrungen im Höhentraining mit Mittelstrecklerinnen. Leistungssport 1986;2:23–25.
11   Lychatz S: Tendenzen der trainingsmethodischen Entwicklung in den Ausdauersportarten im Olympiazyklus 1985 bis 1988, 2. Teil. Leistungssport 1989;6:41–43.
12   Nowacki PE: The physiological bases of high altitude training for improvement of sports performance at sea level. 1988 Seoul Olympic Scientific Congress Organizing Commitee (ed): New Horizons of Human Movement. Seoul, 1988, Abstracts, vol III D9, Sports Physiology, p 181.
13   Shephard RJ: An integrated approach to cardiorespiratory performance at sea level and at an altitude of 7,350 feet; in Cumming GR, Sindal D, Taylor AW (eds): Environmental Effects on Work Performance. Alberta, Printing Services, University of Alberta, 1972, pp 65–86.
14   Faulkner JA: Training for maximum performance at altitude. Int Symp, Albuquerque, 1966, p 88.
15   Faulkner JA, Daniels YT, Balke B: Effects of training at altitude on physical performance capacity. J Appl Physiol 1967;23:85–89.
16   Weidemann H, Roskamm H, Zwecher W, Hummel P, Reindel H: Über die Verminderung der Ausdauerleistungsfähigkeit bei acuter Höhenexposition. Symp, Magglingen, 1966, pp 1–15.
17   Kurenkov GT, Absaljamov TM: Alterations in gaseous exchange of swimmers in medium altitude (2150 m) environment. Symp, Moskow, 1966, pp 49–50.
18   Iliev I, Dimitrova A: On the alterations in the respiratory function of athletes during training at medium altitude (in Bulgarian). Probl Phys Culture 1967;12:236–240.
19   Krastev K, Iliev I, Dimitrova A, Kossev R, Bitchev K, Georgiev I: Functional

investigations during the acclimatization of Bulgarian athletes at altitude, in our country and in Mexico (in Bulgarian). Probl Phys Culture 1968;13:43–48.

20 Asahina K, Ikai M, Ogawa S: A study on acclimatization to altitude in Japanese athletes. Symp, Magglingen, 1966, pp 240–246.

21 Volkov NI, Tcheremissinov VN, Rasumovskii EA: Alterations in specific working capacity of middle and long distance runners during acclimatization and training at an altitude of 2000 m. Symp, Moscow, 1966, p 19.

22 Muchamedjarov TK: A study on the training methods of middle and long distance runners at medium altitude and on the working capacity along the reacclimatization (in Russian). Autoref Diss No. 735, Central Inst Physical Culture, Moscow, 1968, pp 21–25.

23 Murray RH, Shropshire S, Thompson L: Attempted acclimatization by vigorous exercise during periodic exposure to simulated altitude. J Sportsmed Phys Fitness 1968;8:135–143.

24 Farfel VS, Absaljamov TE, Artikov MA, Kurenkov GI, Mironov VI, Tchuparov EA: The parameters of respiration and the working capacity of athletes during exercise at medium altitude; in: Adaptation of Athletes during Exercise at Different Oxygen Regimen (in Russian). Moscow, 1969, pp 8–15.

25 Faulkner JA, Kolias J, Favour CB, Buskirk ER, Balke B: Maximum aerobic capacity and running performance at altitude. J Appl Physiol 1968;24:685–691.

26 Saltin B: Aerobic and anaerobic work capacity at 2300 m. Int Symp, Magglingen, 1966, pp 81–87.

27 Hollman WG: Sport in mittleren Höhen. Sportarzt Sportmed 1966;17:114–122.

28 Drews A: Stoffwechseluntersuchungen bei trainierten während Fahrradergometerbelastungen in mittleren Höhen. Symp, Magglingen, 1966, pp 88–97.

29 Roskamm H, Weidemann H, Samek L, Goernandt L, Baumann A, Mellerowicz H, Renemann H, Limon-Lason R: Maximale Sauerstoffaufnahme, maximales Atemminutenvolumen und maximale Herzfrequenz bei Hochleistungsportlern im Verlaufe einer Akklimatissationsperiode in Font Romeu (1800 m) und Mexico City (2240 m). Sportarzt Sportmed 1968;19:120–133.

30 Owen R, Pugh LGCE: Report of medical research project into effects of altitude in Mexico City in 1965. British Olympic Association, London, 1966.

31 Bierstecker PA, van Leevan AM: Physiological effects of medium altitude (a physiological research project initiated and financed by the Netherlands Olympic Committee and the Netherlands Sport Federation). Asten, Schriks Drukkerij, 1966.

32 Scano A, Dal Monte A, Rossanigo F, Ianigro G: Esplorazione funzionale di atleti italiani prima, durante e dopo cinque settimane di permanenza all 'altidudine di 2250 m; in Scano A, Venerando A (eds): Studi sull' acclimatazione degli atleti italiani a citta del Messico. Roma, CONI, Scuola centrale dello sport, Istituto di medicina dello sport, 1968, pp 31–45.

33 Venerando A: Premières données sur l'acclimatement des athletes italienes à Mexico. Symp, Magglingen, 1966, pp 288–300.

34 Grover RF, Reeves JT: Exercise performance of athletes at sea level and 3100 m altitude. Symp, Magglingen, 1966, pp 130–148.

35 Hughes RL, Clode M, Edwards RHT, Goodwin TJ, Jones NL: Effect of inspired O_2 on cardiopulmonary and metabolic responses to exercise in man. J Appl Physiol 1968; 24:336–347.

36 Artinjuk AA, Bregman MA, Gandelsman AB, Popov SI: On the peculiarity of the intensive exercises at medium altitude; in: Proc 10th Allunion Scientific Conf Physiology, Morphology, Biomechanics and Biochemistry of Muscle Activity, Tbilissy, 1968, vol I, pp 29–30 (in Russian).

37   Reeves JT, Grover RF, Cohn JE: Regulation of ventilation during exercise at 10200 feet
      in athletes born at low altitude. J Appl Physiol 1967;22:546–554.
38   Margaria R, Milic-Emili G, Petit GM, Cavagna R: Mechanical work of breathing
      during muscular exercise. J Appl Physiol 1960;15:354–358.
39   Farfel VS: Respiration at medium altitude and the possibilities of modelling it at sea
      level; in Symp, Alma Ata 1965, pp 91–93.
40   Consolazio CF, Nelson RA, Matoush le Roy O, Hansen JE: Energy metabolism at high
      altitude (3475 m). J Apply Physiol 1966;21:1732–1740.
41   Alipov AD: Some ways to take advantage of the environment at medium altitude in
      Tjan Shjan for sports training. Symp Alma Ata, 1965, pp 11–14.
42   Ivanov NA, Hwan MY: The work of athletes at medium altitude. Symp, Alma Ata,
      1965, pp 42–44.
43   Vogel JA, Harris CW: Cardiopulmonary response of resting man during early exposure
      to high altitude. J Appl Physiol 1967;22:1124–1128.
44   Piiper J, Cerretelli P, Cuttica F, Mangilli F: Energy metabolism and circulation in dogs
      exercising in hypoxia. J. Appl Physiol 1966;21:1143–1149.
45   Donevan RE, Anderson NM, Sekely P, McGregor M: Influence of voluntary hyperven-
      tilation on cardiac output. J Appl Physiol 1962;17:487–491.
46   McGregor M, Donevan RE, Anderson NM: Influence of carbondioxide and hyperventi-
      lation on cardiac output in man. J Appl Physiol 1962;17:933–937.
47   Kontos HA, Levasseur JE, Richard DW, Mauco HP, Paterson JL: Comparative
      circulatory responses to systematic hypoxia in man and in unanasthetized dog. J Appl
      Physiol 1967;23:381–386.
48   Buskirk FR, Kollias J, Akers RF, Prokop FK, Reatigue FP: Maximal performance at
      altitude and on return from altitude in conditioned runners. J Appl Physiol 1967;
      23:259–266.
49   Letunov SP: A study on the process of acclimatization and working capacity of athletes
      at medium altitude. Symp, Moscow, 1966, pp 51–55.
50   Kollias I, Buskirk ER, Akers RF, Prokop K, Baker PT, Reatigue EP: Work capacity of
      long time residents and new commers to altitude. J Appl Physiol 1968;24:792–799.
51   Astrand PO: Circulatory and respiratory response to acute and prolonged hypoxia
      during heavy exercise. Symp, Magglingen, 1966, pp 16–27.
52   Pugh LGCE: Cardiac output in muscular exercise at 5800 m (19000 ft). J Appl Physiol
      1964;19:441–447.
53   Pugh LGCE, Gill MB, Lahiri S, Milleddge JS, Ward MP, West JB: Muscular exercise
      at great altitudes. J Appl Physiol 1964;19:431–440.
54   Lahiri S, Milledge JS, Chattonadhyay HP, Bhattacharyya AK, Linha AK: Respiration
      and heart rate of Sherpa highlanders during exercise. J Appl Physiol 1967;23:545–554.
55   Astrand PO, Rodahl K: Textbook of Work Physiology, New York, McGraw-Hill, 1970,
      pp 159–160.
56   Benesh R, Benesh RE: The effect of organic phosphates from the human erythrocyte on
      the alosteric properties of haemoglobin. Biochem Biophys Res Commun 1967;26:162–
      169.
57   Lenfant C, Torrance JD, Reynafarje C: Shift of the O2-Hb dissociation curve at
      altitude: mechanisms and effect. J Appl Physiol 1971;30:625–629.
58   Reynafarje C: Haematologic changes during rest and physical activity in man at high
      altitude; in Weihe WH (ed): The Physiolgical Effects of High Altitude. Oxford,
      Pergamon Press, 1964, pp 73–81.
59   Krastev K, Iliev I: L'entrainement du sportif dans la haute montagne. Recueil Xe Congr
      FIMS, Belgrad, 1954, pp 74–83.

60   Krastev K, Iliev I, Staikov I: Untersuchungen über Akklimatisation und Training in
     Gebirge. Theorie Praxis Körperkultur 1956;5:713–719.

61   Zima AG, Anishtenko VI, Kan TV, Saralieva SM, Jidkov NV: Efficiency of adaptation
     to intensive sport training at altitude; in Zarifjan AG (ed): The Peculiarity of Sports
     Training at Altitude (in Russian). Frunse, Kirgisian State University, 1987, pp 21–30.

62   Newhouse MT, Becklake MR, Maklem PT, McGregor M: Effect of alterations in end
     tidal CO_2 tension on flow resistance. J Appl Physiol 1964;19:745–749.

63   Hermansen L, Saltin B: Blood lactate concentration during exercise at acute exposure to
     altitude. Symp, Milan, 1966, pp 48–53.

64   Surkina ID, Shioshvilli AP, Merinova AB: Dynamics of adaptability of the respiration
     to exercise at altitude in athletes. Symp Moscow, 1966, pp 75–76.

65   Balke B, Faulkner JA, Daniels IT: Maximum performance capacity at sea level and at
     moderate altitude, before and after training at altitude. Symp, Magglingen, pp 106–116.

66   Iliev I: The importance of the aerobic metabolism in the functional diagnostics in sports
     (in Bulgarian); National Sports Academy, Sofia, 1981.

67   Leith PE, Knuttgen HG, Cymerman A, Feud V, Gabel RA, Steinbrook RA, Steinbrook
     SE: Ventilatory muscle strength and endurance training. J Appl Physiol 1976;41:508–
     516.

68   Robinson EP, Kjeldgaard JM: Improvement in ventilatory muscle function with run-
     ning. J Appl Physiol 1979;46:897–904.

69   Coast JR, Clifford PS, Henrich TW, Stray-Gundersen J, Johnson RL: Inspiratory
     muscle fatigue following maximal exercise. Med Sci Sports, Exercise, 1987, Abstr, vol
     19, p S1.

70   Anholm JD, Stray-Gunderson J, Ramanthan M, Johnson RL: Sustained maximal
     ventilation after endurance exercise in athletes. J Appl Physiol 1989;67:1759–1763.

71   Manohar M: Inspiratory and expiratory muscle perfusion in maximal exercised ponies.
     J Appl Physiol 1990;68:544–548.

72   Powers SK, Lawler J, Criswell D, Dodd S, Grinton S, Bagby G, Silverman H:
     Endurance-training induced cellular adaptations in respiratory muscles. J Appl Physiol
     1990;68:2114–2118.

73   Terrados N, Jansson E, Sylven C, Kaijser L: Is hypoxia a stimulus for synthesis of
     oxidative enzymes and myoglobin? J Appl Physiol 1990;68:2369–2372.

74   Gregs SG, Willis WT, Brooks GA: Interactive effects of anemia and muscle oxidative
     capacity on exercise endurance. J Appl Physiol 1989;67:765–770.

75   Jones NL, Robertson DG, Kane JW, Hart RA: Effect of hypoxia on free fatty acids
     metabolism during exercise. J Appl Physiol 1972;33:733–738.

76   Rowell LB, Saltin B, Kiens B, Christensen NG: Is peak quadriceps blood flow in
     humans even higher during exercise with hypoxemia? Am J Physiol 1986;251:H1038–
     H1044.

77   Bender PR, Groves BM, Cullough RE, McCullough RG, Trad L, Young AJ, Cymer-
     man A, Reeves JT: Decreased exercise muscle lactate release after high altitude acclima-
     tisation. J Appl Physiol 1989;67:1456–1462.

78   Karvonen J, Peltola E, Saarela J: Blood lactate concentration during sprint training
     performed in hypoxic environment. Ann ISEF 1985;4:235–241.

79   Karvonen J, Peltola E, Saarela J: The effect of sprint training performed in a hypoxic
     environment on specific performance capacity. J Sports Med 1986;26:219–224.

80   Karvonen J, Peltola E, Naevery H, Haerkoenen M: Lactate and phosphagen levels in
     muscle immediately after a maximum 300 m run at sea level and at altitude. Res Q Exerc
     Sport 1990;61:108–110.

81a Karvonen J, Essen-Gustavson B, Linderholm H, Peltola E: Influence of sprint training at a moderate altitude on enzyme activities in skeletal muscle of man. Biol Sport 1990;7:153–161.

81b Karvonen J, Peltola E, Saarela J, Niemienen MM: Changes in running speed, blood lactic acid concentration and hormone balance during sprint training performed at an altitude of 1860 m. J Sport Med 1990;30:122–126.

82 Balke B, Daniels JT, Faulkner JA: Training for maximum performance at altitude. Symp, Milan, 1966, pp 179–186.

83 Weihe WH: Time course of adaptation to different altitudes at tissue level. Symp, Magglingen, 1966, pp 177–190.

84 Jensen CR, Fisher AG: Scientific Bases of Athletic Conditioning. Philadelphia, Lea & Febiger, 1979, pp 281–286.

85 Saltin B: The physiological and biochemical basis of aerobic and anaerobic capacities in man: Effect of training and range of adaptation. 2nd Scand Conf Sports Medicine, Oslo, 1986, pp 16–59.

86 Jackson CGR, Sharkey BJ: Altitude, training and human performance. Sports Med 1988;6:279–284.

87 Suslov FP: The Main Problems of Altitude Training of Elite Athletes; in Zarifjan AG (ed): The Pecularity of Sports Training at Altitude (in Russian). Frunse, Kirgisian State University, 1987, pp 98–102.

88 Bishon M: L'antreinement en altitude moyenne. Sport, Bruxelles; 1986; vol 4, pp 44–46.

89 Timushkin AV: the Training of Middle and Long Distance Runners at Different Altitudes; in Zarifjan AG (ed). The Pecularity of Sports Training at Altitude (in Russian). Frunse, Kirgisian State University, 1987, pp 103–109.

Prof. Iltho Iliev, Centre of Applied Research in Sports, 1 N Gabrovsky, Sofia 1172 (Bulgaria)

Karvonen J, Lemon PWR, Iliev I (eds): Medicine in Sports Training and Coaching.
Med Sport Sci. Basel, Karger, 1992, vol 35, pp 104–114

Etiology, General Treatment and Rehabilitation of Sports Injuries

Dimiter Shoilev

Clinic of Sports Traumatology, Sofia, Bulgaria

Contents

Introduction

Over the past few years, a sharp rise in athletic performance levels has been observed in many various sports worldwide. This is to be attributed to extremely vigorous and highly specialized training activities, both in terms of volume and intensity, based on the deliberate incorporation of up-to-date scientific advancements. At the same time, it is worth noting that at the present stage of development, modern athletic training with its specificity and high intensity proves to be a borderline condition between normal human physiology and a number of pathological variations, constantly striving to reach a delicate balance between too much and too little. The balance between these two mutually incompatible processes is an issue of utmost importance, challenging contemporary sports medicine.

The physical and mental status of the individual competitive athlete is controlled by means of a correctly conducted, programmed initial selection process with respect to the acquired knowledge from biomedical studies as well as investigations with a biochemical and functional orientation dealing, with the problems of body conditioning, along with accurate dosing and determination of the maximum physiological threshold of all-out training workloads. Here, adequate physical, medical and mental recovery in the 'workout-to-workout' interval plays a major role. In addition, particularly in cases of early sports specialization, an exceptionally high rate of musculoskeletal injury, resulting in a serious loss of practice days, decline of athletic condition and the occasional complete abandonment of sports is observed. Due to a variety of causes, athletic injuries among persons engaged in recreational sports activities are likewise increasing.

The Problems of Trauma in Modern Sports

It should be pointed out that the various traumatic problems associated with modern sports, of rising incidence and intensity, are characterized by their proper specificity in terms of nature, location, therapeutic approach and recovery. In general, it basically involves traumatic orthopaedic diseases, governed by common mechanisms relating to the occurence and development of the lesion, but essentially differing in terms of specificity, speed of recovery and readaptation.

Inappropriate selection of competitive athletes with respect to various sports events, as well as major errors in the methodology of athletic training (faulty training), are considered to be the underlying causes of sports injuries encountered. Hence, to attain top athletic efficiency only young individuals, endowed with good mental and physical condition and an ideal basic state of health, should be exposed to exhaustive athletic workloads. The aforementioned facts led scientists from various countries worldwide to seek criteria and work out methods for genetic selection of prospective athletes, i.e. to search for youngsters with well defined, specifically oriented psychomotor predisposition for both noncontact (individual) and contact sports (games).

Of all of the possible errors in athletic training methodology which lead to an ever increasing incidence of sports injuries, those listed below are the most frequently encountered and should be given due consideration:

(1) Irregularity in the training, including abrupt changes in the intensity, duration and frequency of training, i.e. maltraining.

(2) Accelerated increase in training workload, especially among teenagers, without due adaptation of the musculoskeletal system.

(3) Failure to make a correct decision concerning the time a convalescent athlete with a history of microtrauma or surgical intervention of varying location and severity is capable of returning to pre-injury activity.

(4) Lack of constant feedback and coordination between coaches and medical personnel involved.

(5) Insufficient awareness on the part of physicians and coaches of the physical qualities and physiological peculiarities of individual competitive athletes.

(6) Inadequate, poor quality selection of competitive athletes.

Adaptation of the musculoskeletal system to increasing workout stress is a process which is fairly continuous and dependent on the level of the theoretical and practical abilities of physicians and coaches on the one hand, and on the constitutional peculiarities of athletes on the other. Any means of accelerating the process may result in adverse traumatic changes in the athletes, mainly of a repetitive microtraumatic nature. Both personal statistical data, and that published by renowned centers specializing in sports injuries (in France, USA, Germany, etc.) point to a noticeable increase in the rate of injuries resulting from overuse of the musculoskeletal system. Sports injuries present a most variegated character, but they also exhibit a certain degree of specificity related to the particular type of sports event. Thus, the pubo-adductor syndrome is usually observed among soccer players, fencers, gymnasts and the like, whenever the lower extremities in the region of the hip joint assume an overstressed position in abduction. A variety of traumatic soft tissue changes in the shoulder joint are recorded among volleyball and handball players, gymnasts, etc. Traumatic changes in the knee and ankle joints affect a vast contingent of competitive athletes. Lately, an increase in traumatic changes involving the spine have also been noted, mainly among weightlifters, wrestlers and gymnasts, etc., occasionally giving rise to serious complications. Owing to the early specialization of athletes, a considerable increase in the number of affections due to aseptic necrosis with diverse location are also observed. New nosological entities, strictly limited to sports injuries, have also emerged, such as the apex patellae syndrome, m. semimembranosus syndrome and the like. Owing to the rich clinical experience in dealing with knee lesions sustained during athletic activities, the past few years have marked a radical increase in our knowledge of knee pathology. According to Trillat [1], 'The philosophy of thinking about the knee joint in terms of functional potentials and stabilizing mechanisms involved have altered our approach to its reconstruction.' Some of the more serious lesions (heavy shaft fractures, fracture-dislocations of the spine, dislocations of large joints and multiple injuries) are relatively seldom seen in athletics, although nowadays their incidence is rising, e.g. motorcycle racing, car racing, downhill skiing, ski jumping and soccer.

The most challenging task facing modern sports traumatology, proceeding from the principles of general traumatology and orthopedics with due consideration to the functional potentialities of the young and physically fit (trained) body, is returning the injured athlete within the shortest possible time to preinjury activity, including routine daily work, as well as exposure to highly demanding training and psychological stresses. This implies making available high level orthopedic and traumatological services, excellent equipment and facilities, and highly educated medical personnel specialized in sports.

Problems Relating to Injuries Resulting from Musculoskeletal Overuse in Sports Activities

Musculoskeletal overuse usually refers to the dynamic stage of a dystrophic or degenerative process involving interstitial spaces and cell elements, developing subsequent to an aseptic inflammatory process resulting in degenerative changes in the following fibrillar structures: tendinous, ligamentous, capsular, muscular, cartilaginous and osseous. In the musculoskeletal system (MSS), exposure to overstress, apart from changes induced by direct mechanical effect, complex trophic disorders of a vasovegatative, metabolic and autogenic character also take place. In other cases, regardless of the motor regimen, there are deviations in the vasovegetative and trophic responses which, under the influence of threshold workloads, give rise to trophic MSS lesions. To gain better insight into the complex interrelations between these factors, we combine them under the mechanical effect heading, i.e. 'aggression', and patterns of the tissue response to such effects under 'biological substrate reaction'. The interrelation between these two basic factors has an essential practical bearing on the course of adaptation or integration with respect to the training level attained and its optimization, overtraining or overfatigue, as well as with respect to the ensuing growth spurt which induces pathological variations in organs and systems, the musculoskeletal system in particular. Viewed in the manner outlined, the problems relating to overuse, overfatigue and overtraining lend themselves well to recovery programming taking into account prophylactic, methodologic, and clinical aspects and areas of expertise with reference to sports training, which is essential in assessing athletic performance efficiency.

Mechanical aggression is produced by a one time exertion, resulting in stratification with ensuing structural disaggregation of the tissue layer. Although the basic symptoms, such as edema, hemorrhage and functional impairment are not infrequently absent, it involves a microtrauma characterized by a quicker than normal course of development. Where systematic effort is involved the example is high-paced repetition, e.g. the contemporary workout routine, where development is characterized by a continuous preliminary period of quantitative accumulations, passing at a given moment into a qualitatively new phase of structural lesion to the region involved. The former type of single effort is usually encountered in younger age groups and above maximum workloads, and may be precluded by proper modelling and well-planned practice sessions for teenagers. Slow development – resulting from the discrepancy between training stress and the adaptation process – is more often seen in mature individuals and competitors of average sports age. Overuse is a process having a cyclic evolutive or involutive character, and at musculoskeletal level it may quickly become chronic owing to reversal of the cause-effect relationship. Such a process could be schematically represented in the form of an ascending spiral, allowing for two-way movement – evolutive and involutive – depending on the interaction of the two basic factors, mechanical aggression and tissue response. Overuse gives rise to sympatheticotonia, leading in turn to vasoconstriction (vascular spasm) which, depending on the local circulation patterns, causes oxygen deficiency and changes in local metabolism associated with a persisting predomination of the dissimilative over assimilative processes – a fact largely implicated in the so-called functional pain occurrence. The prolonged action of dissimilative processes in the tissue leads to development of interstitial edema, assumed to be an expression of an inflammatory process which brings about trophic disorders both within the fibres and at cellular structure level. A degenerative process in its course exerts a deleterious effect on functional fitness and tissue elasticity. Such tissue irritation, apart from the subjective feeling of pain and functional weakness, does under certain conditions of terrain reactivity account for the alteration in the cause-effect relationship, where development of the local degenerative process runs a 'protracted' course even after reducing the training program stress. Gradually, blocking of the interstitium and impairment of the metabolic processes take place until fibrillary structure degeneration of an aseptic type is reached. The processes described are readily apparent at the insertion sites where tendons and ligaments are attached to bones.

Summarizing, the developmental course of overuse diseases of the MSS may be outlined as follows:

(1) Preclinical functional stage where functional vasovegetative disorders and functional pain are predominant.

(2) Stage of clear-cut clinical manifestations with a tendency toward sudden reverse development, 'protracted' course or primary chronification.

(3) Reverse development characterized by complete recovery, with or without subsequent recurrences and secondary chronification.

Chronic interstitial lesions, regardless of apparent repair, are factors contributing to subsequent development of the so-called 'spontaneous' muscle and tendon ruptures. Overuse causes impairment of the kinetic chain, varying in degree with the range of workloads sustained, and with the following anatomohistological characteristics of the tissue: tendon insertion, fascioligamentous insertion, synovio-cartilaginous junction and musculo-tendinous transition. Tendinitis (tendinous, ligamentous and capsular) proves to be the most common lesion encountered in the practice related to sports injuries.

Analysis of the traumatic morbidity rate among sportsmen shows a marked tendency toward increase [2]. Underlying causes of this finding imply persistently increasing stress (in amount and intensity) during the training process, insufficient recovery level, as well as certain drawbacks in the treatment and assessment of athletic fitness and capability as early as the initial stages of the disease.

Role of Cryotherapy in the Treatment of Sports Injuries

Over the last few years, cryotherapy has been applied in sports traumatology as an independent form of treatment, exerting a direct effect on the damaged tissue. Regardless of the fact that the mechanism of the action of cooling has been extensively discussed in the pertinent medical literature, to date no orderly theory has been postulated to explain in a comprehensive manner its physiological effect. Cold applications to the body or muscle gives rise to a number of changes, including raising the irritation threshold of the muscle-fibre pain receptors, decreasing intensity of the metabolic processes, lessening of abnormal muscle tone (spasticity) associated with traumatic lesions and circulation enhancement in the injured zone. There are authors who believe that following cryotherapy, there is not only an absence of a vasodilating effect but, on the contrary, a marked vasoconstricting effect. This is a further confirmation of the fact that research data on the specific mechanism involved in the action of cold is not adequately clarified and conclusive, as is the clinical effect obtained after treatment with ice, such as a pack or massaging block.

The uses of cryotherapy in the management of sports injuries are:

(1) As an initial treatment, instituted immediately after sustaining the injury.

(2) As an integral part of the rehabilitation program.

Local cooling is applied in the form of ice packs, specifically ice compresses. Prior to ice compress application, the injured area is daubed with vaseline or other neutral cream to obviate hazardous local freezing. The compress is held in place for a 15 to 20-min period. During the first 3–4 days after injury, an average of 8–10 procedures are performed. Exercise therapy is carried out immediately after removal of the cryocompresses. Recently, ice massaging has been widely used as an element of rehabilitation in dealing with some athletic injuries, such as sprains, strained muscles and the like, and as a method of prophylaxis as well.

Role of Corticoids in the Treatment of Sports Injuries

Corticoid preparations are endowed with the property of suppressing practically all mesenchymal reactions, i.e. to affect exudative inflammatory and proliferative reactions, as well as to exert antitoxic and immunosuppressive action. These effects explain their wide use and popularity in the treatment of athletic injuries. The most common indications for local administration of corticoid agents include capsuloligamentous lesions, various types of tendinitis, joint adhesions, intermittent hydrarthrosis, postoperative joint effusions, strained articular capsule and the like. Contra-indications include: bacterial infection around the joint, presence of absolute contra-indications for systemic corticoid therapy, susceptibility to bleeding, etc.

The use of corticoid agents is contraindicated in recent tissue lesions because they interfere with the formation of fibroblasts and new capillaries. Their only effect in this case is prompt analgesia, which actually renders them particularly hazardous for application in the practice of traumatology. Following corticoid administration the patient is deprived of his own basic protective barrier – the feeling of pain – and as a result, due to the analgetic effect, the degree of traumatic tissue lesion increases. Instead of local administration of corticoids during this initial, manifest wound phase of the trauma, characterized by the presence of local hematomas, intra-articular effusions, joint function restriction and the like, treatment by cryotherapy, rest and administration of antiphlogistic, analgetic and antiexudative drugs is indicated. In the period characterized by the regenerative process (the first 10–15 postinjury days), local administration of corticoid agents is allowed, provided they do not interfere with the maturation of collagen fibers and their binding into bundles. Local application of corticoids is particularly indicated during the rehabilitation phase. Here, attention should be called to the malpractice and erroneous use of corticoid agents in a variety of pathological conditions of the tendon (tenopathies). Many colleagues resort to local administration of large doses of depot-corticoid agents intratendinously, constantly striving to reach a prompt analgetic effect that allows the injured athlete to return to his daily training activities. Thus, conditions are created promoting the development of intratendinous necrosis with ensuing late degeneration, specifically, tendon ruptures. In our clinical practice, development of numerous ruptures of the

Achilles tendon (soccer, basketball, track and field) and of the long head of the biceps brachii muscle (gymnasts, wrestlers, weightlifters) were observed to coincide with local corticoid therapy.

The various types of corticoid preparations, applied by competent and skilled orthopedic surgeons according to clear indications, yield optimal therapeutic results in a great number of diseases and injuries specific to the practice of sports traumatology. However, their use in cases of misjudgment of the indications, e.g. at an inopportune stage of the disease, involving overdosage, etc., will contribute greatly to the development of a number of irreversible complications of both a topical and systemic nature. It is this unreasonable and incompetent handling of the local administration of corticoid agents that led us to undertake a thorough discussion of the matter and outline our concepts based on many years of clinical experience.

Specificity of Rehabilitation in Sports Injuries

The rehabilitation of injured athletes is based on principles identical to the rehabilitation of any patient presenting musculoskeletal problems, although a certain degree of specificity should be borne in mind, as follows:

(1) Rehabilitation measures for patient-athletes are applied almost immediately after the trauma. Early and properly conducted rehabilitation is of utmost importance for the favorable outcome of treatment.

(2) Before beginning treatment, a thorough assessment of the patient's condition is done – medical, psychological, occupational and social. Professional evaluation has important practical implications in the rehabilitation process. The circumstances in which the injured athlete must return to his individual sports activity after regaining his preinjury condition, particularly within the shortest possible time, with completely restored ability to withstand high-pressure workouts, presents a special challenge in sports rehabilitation. Hence, it follows that the rehabilitation program for athletes has both complex therapeutic and therapeutic-training aspects.

(3) Recovery through a rehabilitation program encompasses a complex of indispensable rehabilitation steps, terms for their realization and members making part of the rehabilitation team.

(4) The work of specialists involved in the restorative process is organized on teamwork basis.

(5) Insofar as rehabilitation is an active process, it follows that the athlete under treatment becomes familiar with the rehabilitation program

from the very beginning; thus, he is appropriately motivated, cooperative, and conscious of the serious demands and specific type of stress with which he is expected to cope.

(6) The rehabilitation process among athletes does not cease with the termination of medical rehabilitation. From the rehabilitation clinic ward where therapeutic-athletic training begins, monitoring of the convalescent athlete by the attending kinesitherapist proceeds within the team environment up to the moment he is capable of fully participating in the training process.

(7) The last, but not least important principle to the rehabilitation of athletic injuries is the close relationship that should be mandatory between the rehabilitation team, coach and sports manager. These interrelationships, based on proper foundations, mutual understanding and assistance, contribute greatly to the success of the overall treatment process.

Apart from the aforementioned basic principles, the rehabilitation approach to injured athletes is characterized by some rather important additional tasks:

(1) Throughout the full period of recovery, general conditioning should be maintained almost equal to the preinjury level.

(2) Using the methods of so-called therapeutic-athletic training, the athlete should be integrated into a workout routine appropriate to the event for which he is training.

General conditioning is incorporated into the earliest rehabilitation measures and proceeds until the athlete returns to his teamwork activities. It is carried out at the hospital bedside, in the gym, swimming pool and the like. All unaffected body parts are exercised with the exception of the area involved. The stress of the training program requires all-out efforts and is based on general athletic training principles. In this manner, after the athlete has undergone medical rehabilitation and is almost functionally fit, and on resuming routine activities in a team setting, he must be ready to be immediately integrated into the normal training process.

The goal of the therapeutic-athletic training program is to reintroduce the body part affected (usually upper or lower limb) to the normal workout routine. It is integrated into the final stage of the rehabilitation program, i.e. when the level of functional recovery attained allows exposure to physical exertions, specific to the individual sports event. First, only elements of the sports event practiced are included, followed by drills involving movements and skills most characteristic of the respective sports discipline. The implementing of the therapeutic-athletic practice program implies a strictly individual approach and invariably begins within the framework of medical rehabilitation; subsequently, sessions are conducted with the team under the supervision of the kinesitherapist. Thereafter, when the condition of the athlete allows, and after consulting the attending physician, the patient is put under the charge of the coach for exposure to high-pressure stress.

In operative treatment of athletic injuries, rehabilitation usually begins during the preoperative period, proceeds at the bedside from the second postoperative day where, in conjunction with exercise therapy, general conditioning techniques are also employed. Later, the therapeutic sessions are conducted in the gym where exposure to heavier workloads is possible, utilizing variable resistance-exercise equipment. Physical therapy procedures are also added with regard to the local therapeutic effect, and prophylaxis against postoperative complications, such as Sudeck's atrophy and joint contractures. In the final stage of the general rehabilitation program, so-called therapeutic-athletic training is incorporated as one of the basic elements in the recovery of injured athletes.

Obviously, rehabilitation of injured athletes, unlike that in ordinary patients, has a number of essential peculiarities. Differences stem mainly from the fact that the athlete should regain a fitness level enabling him to perform not only daily living and working activities, but also to endure the highly demanding physical exertions associated with modern sports, i.e. there is an essential difference between 'health' in normal life, and 'health' in professional sports. This places a great responsibility on persons facing problems relating to athletic recovery including physicians, physical therapists and coaches.

Conclusion

Inappropriate selection of competitive athletes with respect to various sports events as well as major errors in the methodology of athletic training (faulty training) are considered to be the underlying causes of sports injuries encountered. Hence, to attain top athletic efficiency only young individuals, endowed with good mental and physical condition and an ideal basic state of health, should be exposed to exhaustive athletic workloads. Musculoskeletal overuse usually refers to the dynamic stage of a dystrophic or degenerative process involving interstitial spaces and cell elements, developing subsequent to an aseptic inflammatory process resulting in degenerative changes in the following fibrillar structures: tendinous, ligamentous, capsular, muscular, cartilaginous and osseous. Over the last few years, cryotherapy has been applied in sports traumatology as an independent form of treatment, exerting a direct effect on the damaged tissue. Cold application to the body or muscle gives rise to a number of changes, including raising the irritation threshold of the muscle fiber pain receptors, decreasing intensity of the metabolic processes, lessening of abnormal muscle tone (spasticity) associated with traumatic lesions and circulatory enhancement in the injured zone. The corticoid preparations are endowed with the property of suppressing practically all mesenchymal reactions, i.e. to affect exudative inflammatory and proliferative reactions, as well as to exert antitoxic and immunosuppressive action. Following corticoid administration, the patient is deprived of his own basic protective barrier – the feeling of pain – and as a result, due to the analgetic effect, the degree of traumatic tissue lesion increases. The rehabilitation of injured athletes is based on principles identical to the rehabilitation of any patient presenting musculoskeletal problems, although a certain degree of specificity should be borne in mind. Early and properly conducted rehabilitation is of utmost importance for the favourable outcome of treatment.

References

1   Trillat A: Rev Chir Orthop 1972;(Suppl I):111.
2   Shoilev D: Sports Traumatology. Sofia, Medicina i. Fizkultura, 1983.

Dimiter Shoilev, Clinic of Sports Traumatology, Diana 2, Sofia (Bulgaria)

Karvonen J, Lemon PWR, Iliev I (eds): Medicine in Sports Training and Coaching.
Med Sport Sci. Basel, Karger, 1992, vol 35, pp 115 159

Heart Rate Monitoring for Estimation of Training Intensity

Peter G.J.M. Janssen

Sportmedische Praktijk Deurne, The Netherlands

Contents

Introduction

For athletes it is important to know how to gain maximum benefits from training. Therefore, it is necessary to understand how the body functions during physical exercise. Unfortunately, many athletes and even their coaches frequently have inadequate training in exercise science. This often produces less than optimal benefits from physical training. Training workouts can be too intensive leading to a state of over-training and/or an increased prevalence of sports related injuries or not intense enough producing inadequate levels of preparation. High quality training will not only benefit the elite performer but the recreational athlete as well. The present article deals with various forms of training based on the underlying physiological principles. It discusses how to train using heart rate (HR or pulse rate, PR) and how to analyse HR records of races and workouts.

Basic Principles

Energy Supply during Exercise

There are several energy-supplying systems [1–3] and each system can be trained separately. A central place in energy supply is taken by a chemical substance which enables muscles to contract. This substance is called adenosine triphosphate (ATP). It is a compound which is broken down to adenosine diphosphate (ADP) during muscular activity. The process supplies the muscle with its energy. Schematically, this process may be presented as follows:

$$ATP \rightarrow ADP + \text{inorganic phosphate} + \text{energy}.$$

The quantity of ATP in the muscles is very limited and if not regenerated would be exhausted in only a few seconds of intense exercise.

Fortunately, in the muscle there are a number of systems which regenerate ATP from the ADP thus produced so that the quantity of ATP remains constant and the muscle can keep on contracting for 5–8 s.

ADP + phosphopcreatine (PC) → ATP + creatine.

The systems that become important in ATP regeneration after these 5–8 s use the oxidation reaction with oxygen of foodstuffs, i.e. carbohydrates, fats and protein. These carbohydrates, fats and protein are consumed in the everyday meals. The magnitude of restored fat is nearly unlimited; however, the quantity of carbohydrates, e.g. sugars, starches and glycose stored as glycogen mainly in the liver and muscles is relatively small. This store can vary widely (as a result of prior diet and exercise) but as a rule it is sufficient for at least 1 h of maximum performance. Protein is a minor energy fuel because it is not stored for energy but rather plays a structural or functional (enzymatic) role in the body.

The break down of fats occurs as follows:

Fats + oxygen + ADP → carbon dioxide + ATP + water.

The break down of carbohydrates involves two steps.

1st step:

Glucose + ADP → lactate + ATP.

The first step can occur without lactate formation.

2nd step:

Lactate + oxygen + ADP → carbon dioxide + ATP + water.

The second step can utilize pyruvate.

The first step (anaerobic glycolysis) does not use oxygen whereas the second does. When the exercise is not too intense the by-product lactate (also called lactic acid) is directly worked into the second step so that the final result is:

Glucose + oxygen + ADP → carbon dioxide + ATP + water.

As exercise intensity increases the second step cannot keep up with the first one resulting in an accumulation of lactic acid in the exercising muscles.

Characteristics of an increasing acidosis are: sore legs (for the cyclist or runner) or sore arms (for a rower) and a feeling of powerlessness.

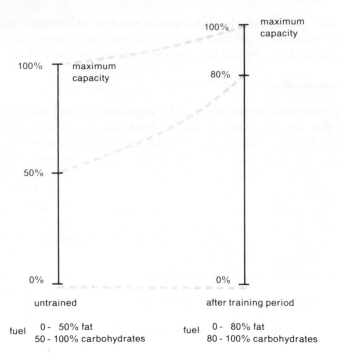

fuel 0 - 50% fat
      50 - 100% carbohydrates

fuel 0 - 80% fat
      80 - 100% carbohydrates

Fig. 1. Effect of amount of training on development of performance capacity and overtraining.

Therefore, the exercise cannot be maintained at the same intensity. In competitions whenever a cyclist or runner must allow a gap between him and the race leader acidosis in the muscles is most likely to be the cause. The athlete who can postpone the moment of acidosis best will mostly likely win the race.

Anaerobic glycolysis is no more than an emergency solution. The resulting acidosis also has several other negative effects, which will be dealt with later (fig. 1).

Survey of the energy-supplying systems:

(a) (i) $ATP \rightarrow ADP + energy$,
    (ii) $ADP + PC \rightarrow ATP + creatine$;
(b) $Glucose + ADP \rightarrow lactic\ acid,\ carbon\ dioxide + ATP$;
(c) $Glucose + oxygen + ADP \rightarrow water,\ carbon\ dioxide + ATP$;
(d) $Fat + oxygen + ADP \rightarrow water + carbon\ dioxide + ATP$;
(e) $Amino\ acids + oxygen + ADP \rightarrow water + carbon\ dioxide + urea + ATP$.

Table 1. Classification of maximum activity of various duration together with energy-supplying system for this activity

Duration	Classification (aerobic/anaerobic)	Energy supplied by	Observations
120–140 s	aerobic + anaerobic,	muscle glycogen	decreasing lactate
1–4 s	anaerobic, alactic	ATP	
4–20 s[1]	anaerobic, alactic	ATP + CP	
20–45 s[1]	anaerobic, alactic +anaerobic, lactic	ATP + CP + muscle glycogen	high lactate production
45–120 s	anaerobic, lactic	muscle glycogen	with increasing duration, decreasing lactate production
120–140 s	aerobic + anaerobic, lactic	muscle glycogen	ditto
240–600 s	aerobic	muscle glycogen +fatty acids	with increasing duration higher share of fats

[1] Some data indicate lactic acid is produced during the first 10 s of intense activity.

Table 2. Various substrates for energy supply and their characteristics

Substrate	Breakdown	Availability	Speed of energy production
Creatine phosphate	anaerobic, alactic	very limited	very fast
Glycogen or glucose	anaerobic, lactic	limited	fast
Glucose or glycogen	aerobic, alactic	limited	slow
Fatty acids	aerobic, alactic	unlimited	sluggish

Characteristics of the Various Energy-Supplying Systems (Table 1–3)
System A: The phosphate battery:
(i) $ATP \rightarrow ADP +$ energy; (ii) $ADP + CP \rightarrow ATP +$ creatine.

This system immediately supplies energy via the ATP present in the muscle cells. The quantity of ATP is, at maximum pace, rapidly exhausted (5–8 s). The supply of energy by breaking down ATP takes place at the onset of the exercise. The phosphate battery is trained by power bursts alternated with periods of rest, because the re-formation of the ATP takes

Table 3. Characteristics of the various energy-supplying systems.

Energy supply	Anaerobic, alactic	Anaerobic, lactic	Aerobic, alactic
Energy via	ATP/CP	glycolysis	burning with oxygen
Yields	direct energy	2–3 mM ATP	36 mM ATP
Time	10 s	15 s to 2 or 3 min	longer than 2–3 min
By-product	no lactate	lactate	no lactate
Name	phosphate battery	lactic system	aerobic system
Activity	start of exertion, sprint	breakaway, brief exertion	long-lasting exertion
Examples	100-meter sprint	closing a gap, 1 km cycling time trial, 400–800 m running	endurance cycling, marathon, long distances
Capacity	sprinting capacity	lactate tolerance capacity	endurance capacity

time. The energy supply via the phosphate battery is alactic (without producing lactid acid) and anaerobic (without using oxygen).

System B: Glycolysis – Glucose + ADP → lactic acid + ATP.

This is an emergency system which accelerates when a certain exercise intensity is surpassed. This intensity varies from individual to individual. Whenever this system becomes the predominant energy supplier the exercise can only continue for a short time (a few minutes at most).

After stopping the exercise it may be some 20–30 min before all the lactic acid in the body is neutralised; high concentrations of lactate give a feeling of tiredness, sore muscles, heavy breathing and a willingness to stop the exercise. Energy supply via this system is anaerobic and lactic.

System C + D: Aerobic system – Glucose or
fat + O_2 + ADP → H_2O + CO_2 + ATP.

System E: Amino acids + O_2 + ADP → H_2O + CO_2 + urea + ATP.

These aerobic energy systems need some time to become maximally activated (2–3 min) and carbohydrate and fat are most important exercise energy sources. The store of carbohydrates can be exhausted in one exercise

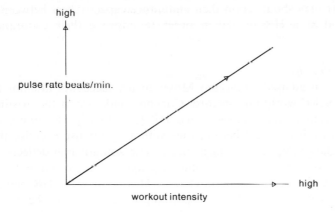

pulse rate beats/min.

workout intensity → high

Fig. 2. See text.

bout while the store of fats is practically unlimited. Exercise of low intensity uses predominantly fat as an energy supplier; however, as the intensity is increased the oxidation of carbohydrates plays a greater and greater role. When the athlete's condition improves fat oxidation continues at higher exercise intensity, thus sparing carbohydrates (fig. 1). These aerobic systems respond very well to training programs regardless of age. Capacity improvements by a factor 50 have been described. Energy supply via this system is aerobic and alactic: Aerobic = using oxygen; anaerobic = without using oxygen; lactic = producing lactic acid; alactic = without producing lactic acid.

Heart Rate and Physical Exercise

In everyday training HR is often used to assess the intensity of the work-out [2–8]. The reason for using HR as a standard of exertion is the discovery that there is a linear correlation between HR and exercise intensity (fig. 2).

For endurance training, the best training stimulus is obtained at an intensity at which the oxygen transport system is activated to the maximum, while lactate accumulation in the muscles is not yet reached. This intensity range is also called the aerobic-anaerobic transit zone between the aerobic and anaerobic threshold.

Many endurance work-outs are done at a HR of about 180 beats per minute. Relative to the aerobic and anaerobic transit zone, this training intensity is usually too high; however, the aerobic and anaerobic threshold varies widely from person to person. Generally, the aerobic-anaerobic transit zone lies within a HR range of 140 and 180 beats per minute.

Therefore, sportsmen should train their endurance capacity best between a HR of 140 and at a HR of 180 in order to improve their endurance capacity.

Conconi's Principle

Prof. Conconi advised Francesco Moser in his successful attempt to break Eddy Merckx' world-hour-record. Conconi made use of the existing correlation between exercise intensity and HR [5, 6, 9–12]. He found, as other investigators had found before, that with very intense exercise the HR/intensity relationship is no longer linear. The straight line deflects at high intensities. In other words: the intensity may be increased but the increase of HR lags at a certain point (fig. 3). This point is the HR deflection point. The exercise intensity corresponding to this point is the maximum activity that can be done with aerobic energy supply. The deflection in the curve marks the HR or exercise intensity (e.g. the speed of running or cycling) beyond which the athlete obtains a large amount of energy via anaerobic pathways. In this way, Conconi could exactly establish the speed that Moser had to maintain without getting exhausted prematurely.

The deflection point marks the maximum speed that can be maintained for a long period of time. It is the highest speed or HR that can be supported aerobically. If the speed is increased further an accumulation of lactate will occur. In this situation, the aerobic energy supplying system does not suffice; the anaerobic system is called upon with the result an increasing accumulation of lactate. In fact, the anaerobic system is engaged earlier but at this point the balance between lactate production and lactate elimination is disturbed in such a way that lactate accumulation sets in rapidly. A great advantage of Conconi's method is that taking blood samples is not necessary. Therefore this method is also called: the bloodless method of establishing the deflection point.

Influence of Endurance Training on Heart Rate

After a period of endurance training the HR response to the same level of exertion changes.

Maximum Exercise Heart Rate

In the example (fig. 4) the untrained athlete has a maximum HR of 200 beats per minute. In general, maximum HR does not depend on conditioning; however, in very well-trained endurance athletes maximum HR may be slightly lower. This may be because maximal cardiac output is reached at submaximal HR.

The maximum HR can only be established when the athlete is fully

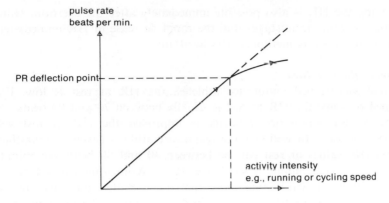

Fig. 3. See text.

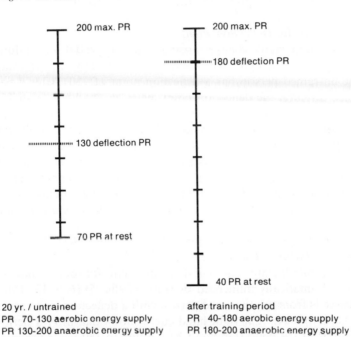

20 yr. / untrained
PR 70-130 aerobic energy supply
PR 130-200 anaerobic energy supply

after training period
PR 40-180 aerobic energy supply
PR 180-200 anaerobic energy supply

Fig. 4. See text.

rested. A complete recovery after the previous work-out is necessary. It is established as follows:

After a warm-up period of some 15 min, the athlete does an all out 5 min of running or cycling. The last 20–30 s are sprinted. The maximum HR can now simply be read on the HR meter.

Counting the HR is also possible immediately after the exertion. However, due to counting mistakes and the rapid decrease in HR immediately after the exertion this method is less accurate.

Heart Rate at Rest

Four well-trained endurance athletes, the HR at rest is low. For untrained persons, the HR at rest is usually between 70 and 80 beats per minute. As the endurance capacity is improved the HR at rest will gradually decrease. In well-training endurance athletes (cyclists, marathon runners) HR values at rest can be between 40 and 50 beats per minute (under 40 beats per minute is sometimes seen). Women have a HR at rest of about 10 beats per minute more than men of the same age. In the morning, HR is about 10 beats per minute less than in the same situation in the evening. This also applies for the maximum HR.

Heart Rate at the Deflection Point

The most important change arising after a period of endurance training is a shift of the deflection point to a higher HR. In the example (fig. 4), the untrained person has a deflection point of 130. After a period of endurance training, the deflection point increases (perhaps from 130 to 180 beats per minute). An intensity beyond the HR of the deflection point will produce an accumulation of lactate. This means that in well-trained endurance athletes the HR range (exercise intensity), where the energy supply is completely aerobic, increases dramatically. As a result the athlete can maintain an endurance exertion for longer and at a higher pace. The athlete has more stamina. Only at very great exercise intensities is the anaerobic system fully activated. As a result, there is less lactate accumulation.

Heart Rate-Lactate Acid Curve

The heart rate-lactate acid curve is different for every individual. Further, it is dramatically influenced by training (fig. 5) [6, 9, 13–15]. The left-hand curve is from an untrained person with a deflection point at a HR of 130 beats per minute. The right hand curve shows that after a period of training the HR at the deflection point has shifted to 180 beats per minute.

The untrained person has great difficulty maintaining exercise at a HR above 130. In contrast, a trained athlete can exercise for a long time at a HR 180. This intensity of exertion roughly corresponds with a blood lactate concentration of 4 mmol/l. The 4 mmol/l threshold is in fact an oversimplification of the relationships between lactate accumulation and relative exercise intensity. The important point is to find out the inflection point of the individual lactate curve on the plot: lactate concentration

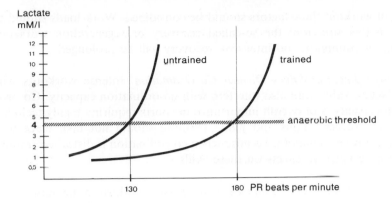

Fig. 5. See text.

versus relative exercise intensity. This inflection point may or may not correspond to 4 mmol/l, depending on factors other than exercise intensity, but it will represent the individual maximum tolerable exercise intensity for endurance training or competition. This individual threshold may further serve as a basis for comparisons with HR in order to estimate the physiological strain during training or competition. The 4 mmol/l value may be misleading in some particular cases despite the fact that it is well established as a statistical mean value for large groups of athletes.

Disadvantageous Effects of Lactate Acid

High lactate concentrations cause an acidosis on and around muscle cells. This acid environment may seriously interfere with various mechanisms in the muscle cells. The acrobic enzymes system in the muscle cell may be seen as a factory plant where aerobic energy supply takes place. This enzyme system is sabotaged by acidosis and as a result aerobic endurance capacity is reduced. It may be days before this system has sufficiently recovered and aerobic capacity is at its old level again [3, 12, 16–19].

When the workload is repeatedly too intense, i.e. without sufficient time to recover, a considerable decrease in aerobic endurance capacity is inevitable. These overly intensive exercise bouts can lead to a complex of complaints known as overtraining. Further, acidosis can cause damage to the muscle cell wall. This causes leakage from the muscle cells into the blood, e.g. increased urea and CK.

It may be 24–96 h before these values have returned to normal again. Recovery of the muscle damage may take a long time. When choosing a form of workout these factors should be considered. Work-loads should be light in this situation: the so-called recovery or regeneration work-out. Whenever training is too intensive, recovery will be prolonged.

High Lactate Values Disturb Co-Ordination. Intense workouts with high lactate values can also interfere with co-ordination capacity. Co-ordination capacity is of overall importance in sports requiring highly technical skills, i.e. soccer, tennis and judo. Training should not take place with lactate above 6–8 mmol/l, because when co-ordination is disturbed training could have negative effects on these skills.

High Lactate Values Enhance Injury Risks. Acidosis in the muscles can lead to microruptures in the muscular tissues. This minor damage may, if insufficiently healed, result in more serious injuries.

The Phosphate System is Disturbed by High Lactate Values. The reformation of ATP is also delayed in acid muscles. Therefore, it is best to avoid high lactate values during sprint training.

Fat Oxidation is Inhibited at High Lactate Values. When glycogen reserves are depleted energy supply is endangered at high lactate values because fat oxidation is inhibited.

Training

Energy-Supplying Systems and Their Meaning to
Various Forms of Training
Every sport has its own specific forms of training, i.e. a marathon runner trains differently from a sprinter. The former will especially train to develop a large endurance and aerobic capacity, whereas the sprinter will be very interested in having an excellently trained anaerobic capacity [1, 12, 18–25].

Some sports performances, e.g. 400 m running, require training of the lactate system. The 400 m runner must learn to fight against the strong acidification of his muscles and the feeling of fatigue that goes along with it. In so doing, he trains his lactate tolerance. The aerobic endurance capacity can best be trained by endurance workouts, i.e. exertions lasting from at least 10 min to half an hour which are done at the same submaximal level. This level may very accurately be established and it is characterized by the fact that an accumulation of lactate does not yet arise.

An increase of the general anaerobic capacity can also be trained of course. An increase of high-energy phosphates is possible with submaximal interval work, the intensity being 80–90% of the maximum. These must be workloads with a duration of 10–20 s followed by a pause long enough to prevent high lactate accumulations in the body. The duration of the pause is 1–3 min, depending on the state of conditioning of the athlete.

If the lactate system is to be trained, the duration of the submaximal training period should be lengthened to some 1–3 min. The short recovery pause must not be so long that the lactate concentration in the blood strongly declines. This means recovery pauses of about 30 s to some minutes depending on the state of conditioning of the athlete. Training of the lactate system as far as necessary may best be done in the form of competition. It should be remembered, however, that two intense races with 1 week's interval may be too much. Such heavy workloads must always be followed by light workouts, the so-called recovery runs. Blood lactate concentration can be measured and it is usually expressed in mmol/l. Healthy persons at rest should have values between 1 and 2 mmol/l. Performing at high levels may lead to an increase of lactate concentration as mentioned. In order to prevent excessive accumulation a lactate workload can be established (fig. 6). Figure 6 indicates the relation between blood lactate concentration and training intensity (running speed).

A lactate workload curve may be obtained by having the athlete run a certain route and then measuring the blood lactate value after every run. Every lap should be run at a constant pace and every new lap should be a little faster than the previous one. The distance run should be such that it can be done in at least 5 min.

In well-trained athletes, low speeds produce low lactic acid values because the demand for energy can completely be met aerobically. As the workload becomes more intense the curve begins to go up, the working muscles produce more lactate, but the quantities are such that they can be neutralized elsewhere in the body.

This is said to be the case with lactate concentrations between 2 and 4 mmol/l. This area is also called the aerobic-anaerobic transit zone. There is a certain pace which may be maintained for a long time without lactate accumulations in the body. If this pace is surpassed a growing acidification will take place and eventually the athlete will be forced to stop. The pace before lactate accumulates is known as the anaerobic threshold. In practice, this is assumed to be at a lactate value of 4 mmol/l because this value approaches the real threshold rather well. So performances over this limit pace lead to an increase of lactate in the body. A graph (fig. 8) should be drawn up for each individual athlete, and used to guide his training.

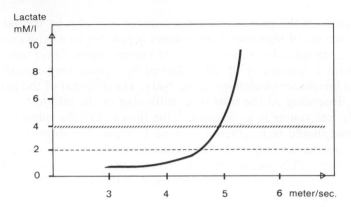

Fig. 6. See text.

It is known that stamina can best be trained by endurance training around the level of the anaerobic lactate threshold, i.e. training paces corresponding with lactate values of 2, 3, 4 and 5 mmol/l. Very well-trained athletes train their endurance capacity at somewhat lower lactate values, usually between 2 and 3 mmol/l while less well-trained persons improve their endurance capacity at somewhat higher values, around 3, 4 and 5 mmol/l lactate.

Recovery runs should keep lactate concentrations lower than 2 mmol/l lactate. Intense interval workouts give high lactate values (far higher than 4 mmol/l lactate). Under the influence of training the curve will shift to the right (fig. 7).

Curves A and B come from the same athlete. Curve A at the beginning of a training period. Curve B at the end of a training period of 3 months. Conclusion: running pace at lactate 4 mmol/l has clearly increased. Curve A 3 m/s against curve B 5 m/s. The curve has shifted to the right. Aerobic capacity has clearly improved. Training intensity must therefore be readjusted every so often. To do so new blood samples must then be taken and unfortunately not every one can obtain repeated blood samples from their athletes.

Lactate Curves of Various Athletes

Figure 8 shows lactate curves of various athletes, all of them well-trained. Every individual has his own curve and the interindividual differences often turn out to be very large. When the athlete with the most right hand curve trains together with the athlete of the left hand curve and the two of them are told to perform at a heart rate of 150 beats per minute, the

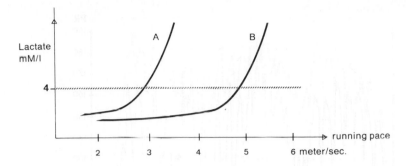

Fig. 7. Curves A and B come from the same athlete. Curve A at the beginning of a training period. Curve B at the end of a training period of 3 months. Conclusion: running pace at lactate 4 has clearly gone up. Curve A 3 m/s against curve B 5 m/s. The curve has shifted to the right. Aerobic capacity has clearly improved.

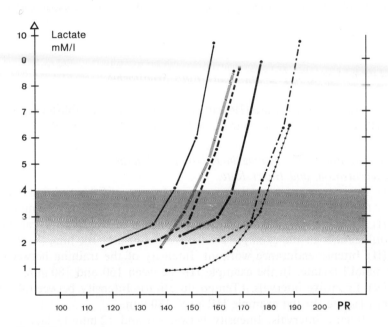

Fig. 8. See text.

left hand curve athlete is going through a very intense workout with high lactate values, whereas the right hand curve athlete hardly exerts himself. For this reason training intensity should be set individually. When training in groups the training task has different effects on different athletes (fig. 8, 9).

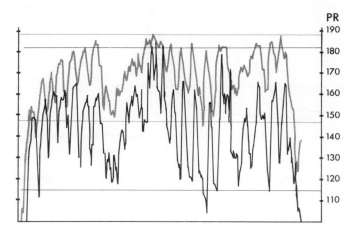

Fig. 9. HR curves of 2 persons of the same age who do the same workout together.

Individual Coaching Using Heart Rate Monitoring

Starting from the lactate-HR curve, it is possible to establish exactly at what HR an athlete should train [2, 4, 6, 18, 19, 23–25] (fig. 10).

Various Forms of Training in Relation to Lactate Concentration and Heart-Rate

(I) Recovery or regeneration workout. Intensity of this training is well under 2 mmol/l lactate. In the example HR between 110 and 140/min.

(II) Extensive endurance workout. Intensity of this training around 2 mmol/l lactate. In the example HR between 140 and 160 min.

(III) Intense endurance workout. Intensity of the training between 3 and 4 mmol/l lactate. In the example HR between 160 and 180 min.

(IV) Extensive intervals. (Tempo duration): Intensity between 4 and 6 mmol/l lactate. In the example HR over 180 min.

(V) Intense intervals. Intensity between 6 and 12 mmol/l lactate. In the example HR over 180 min.

Concepts of Extensive and Intensive Training

Optimal Training of Endurance Capacity. With the help of HR, the intensity of endurance training can be set optimally there by maximizing the benefits of training. By optimizing training it may even be possible to improve performance with less training.

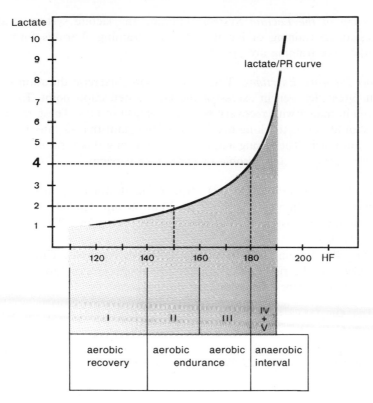

Fig. 10. The various training forms in relation to lactate concentration and HR. (I) Recovery of regeneration workout. Intensity of this training well under 2 mM lactate. In the example between HR 110 and 140. (II) Extensive endurance workout. Intensity of this training around 2 mM lactate. In the example HR between 140–160. (III) Intensive endurance workout. Intensity of the training between 3 and 4 mM lactate. In the example HR between 160–180. (IV) Extensive repetitions (tempo duration). Intensity between 4 and 6 mM lactate. In the example over HR 180. (V) Intensive repetitions (intensive repetitions). Intensity between 6 and 12 mM lactate. In the example HR over 180.

Optimal Training of the Phosphate System. Intense forms of training (such as training the phosphate system and lactate system) can also be optimized with the help of heart rates.

When training the phosphate system the following points should be remembered. The duration of the load is short, viz. 5–10 or 20 s at the most. The intensity is high, being 80–90% of the maximum.

The recovery periods are long (1 min or even longer when necessary). Lactate content should not surpass 6 mmol/l during this workout. The aim of this training is an increase in the quantity of phosphates such as ATP.

Training of the Lactate System. Training the lactate system is also called resistance training or lactate tolerance training. Various forms of lactate tolerance training are possible.

Short Intensive Exertions. This involves short exercise duration (15–180 s) at intensities well in excess of the lactate deflection point. Exercise bouts are alternated with recovery periods from 30 to 60 s. These recovery periods should not be too long because it is important that lactate does not decrease too much. The strong acidosis arising during this form of training may cause damage to the aerobic or endurance capacity.

Long Intense Exertions. In this form of lactate tolerance training the duration of the exertion may be some 20, 30 or 60 min. The intensity of the exercise should be just over the lactate deflection point. There are no recovery periods.

During this training lactate content surpasses 6 mmol/l. This form of training also has the risk of causing damage to endurance capacity. This type of training can best be completed during races (fig. 11, 12).

Examples of Heart Rate Recordings from Practice

Team Time Trial of a 23-Year-Old Professional Cyclist

Test data:

    Lactate 2 = HR 165
    Lactate 3 = HR 175
    Lactate 4 = HR 180

    Maximum HR = 197 (fig. 13)

The recordings were made during a team trial, in Paris, during the Tour de France, 1986. The first part is the warm-up. During the race, until 55 min, he performs well over the level of L4 = HR 180.

The maximum HR reached in the race is 197. After 55 min, he cannot keep up with his teammates any more. At this point he has reached maximum acidosis and therefore cannot follow the pace of the team. Yet he keeps performing up to his limits in order to finish in time. If he should not succeed in this he is out of the race. In spite of the fact that, subjectively, he exerts himself maximally his HR goes down and so does his cycling speed. So he has been overexerting himself above the deflection point. The curve clearly shows that well-trained athletes can perform high in the anaerobic range for long period of time.

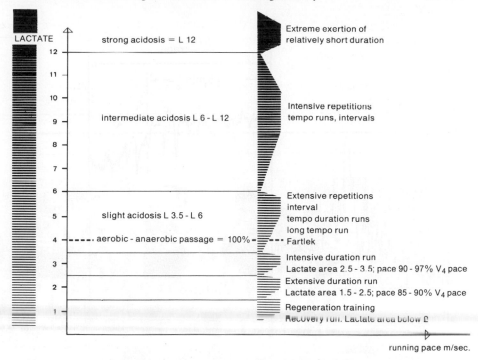

Fig. 11. The various forms of training in relation to lactate concentration and running pace.

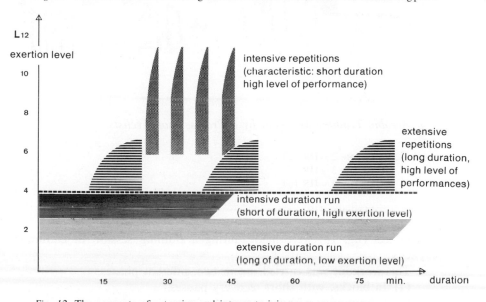

Fig. 12. The concepts of extensive and intense training.

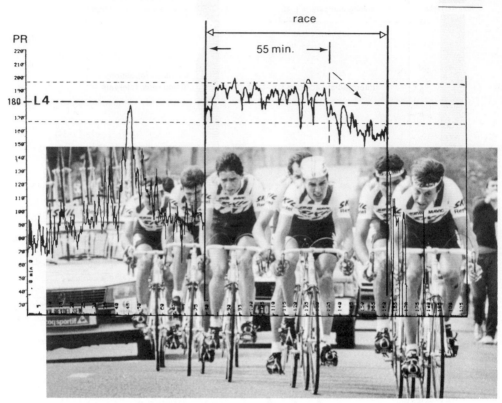

Fig. 13. See text.

Aerobic Training Workout by a Professional Cyclist

Test data: Lactate 2 = HR 150
Lactate 3 = HR 155
Lactate 4 = HR 160

Maximum HR = 175

Recordings (fig. 14) were made during a training session of endurance capacity.

This workout was carried out in two different phases:
(1) In blocks, with short recovery pauses.
(2) Continuous, without recovery pauses.

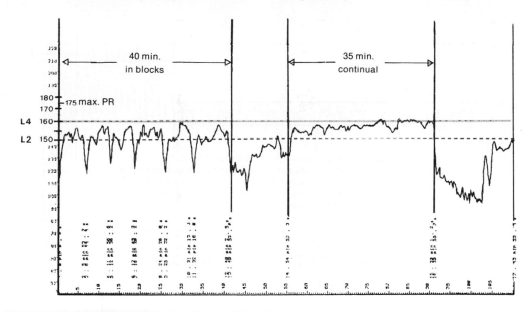

Fig. 14. See text.

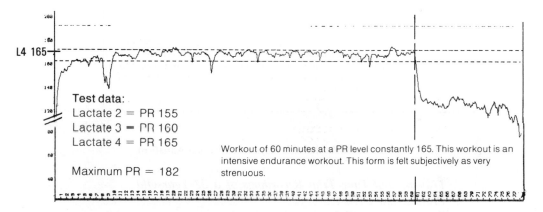

Test data:
Lactate 2 = PR 155
Lactate 3 = PR 160
Lactate 4 = PR 165

Maximum PR = 182

Workout of 60 minutes at a PR level constantly 165. This workout is an intensive endurance workout. This form is felt subjectively as very strenuous.

Fig. 15. Intense endurance workout.

Interpretation:

Correct training of the aerobic system. During the exercise parts, both the blocks and the continuous part, HR is between 150/min and 160/min, so also between L2 and L4.

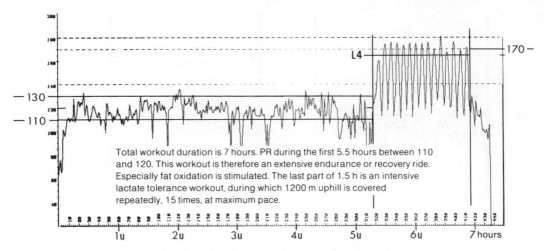

Fig. 16. Combination of endurance and lactate tolerance workout.

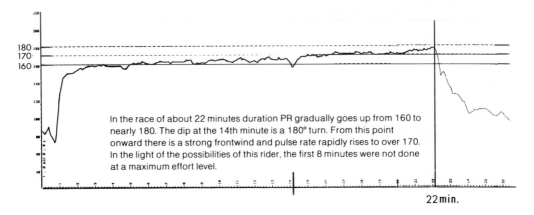

Fig. 17. 14-kilometer time trial in a stage race (Tirreno-Adriatico).

Training and Time Trial Recordings of a 22-Year-Old Professional Cyclist
See figures 15–17 for complete details.

Extensive Endurance Workout of a Triathlete

Test data: Lactate 2 = HR 145

              Lactate 3 = HR 160

              Lactate 4 = HR 170

              Maximum HR = 180

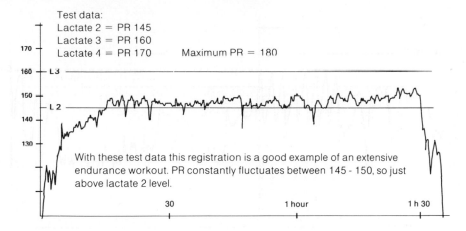

Test data:
Lactate 2 = PR 145
Lactate 3 = PR 160
Lactate 4 = PR 170   Maximum PR = 180

With these test data this registration is a good example of an extensive endurance workout. PR constantly fluctuates between 145 - 150, so just above lactate 2 level.

Fig. 18. See text.

This record (fig. 18) is a good example of an extensive endurance workout. HR constantly fluctuates between 145 and 150 beats per minute, and lactate concentration just above 2 mmol/l.

Interpretation: correct extensive endurance workout.

Sprint Workouts of a Professional Cyclist

Test data: Lactate 2 = HR 150
Lactate 3 = HR 155
Lactate 4 = HR 160

Maximum HR = 175

Task:

A warm-up followed by a sprint workout.
Exertion phases are 10–20 s.
Recovery pauses are long, 3–5 min
HR gradually goes up to maximum HR. (fig. 19a and b)

Interpretation:

HR does not surpass 160. Probably the rider had insufficiently recovered from the previous workout. The recovery pauses are too short. During

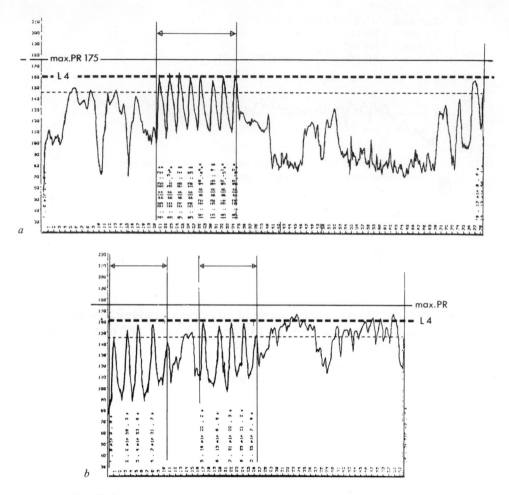

Fig. 19a, b. See text.

sprint workouts high lactate concentrations should be avoided, so recovery pauses must be long. Sprint workouts are only beneficial when complete recuperation has taken place.

During sprint workouts HR goes up somewhat higher with every sprint. Eventually maximum HR should be reached. In these curves maximum HR is not reached.

Aerobic Training Workout by a Professional Cyclist

Test data: Lactate 2 = HR 150
            Lactate 3 = HR 155
            Lactate 4 = HR 160

Maximum HR = 175

The task (fig. 20) was an aerobic workout first in intermittent blocks and then at a continuous pace.

During the short exertion blocks (duration 1–2 min), HR rises to 160 beats per minute and goes down to 120 beats per minute during the short recovery pauses.

During the continuous pace, without recovery breaks (30 min duration) HR is between 150 and 160/min.

The first part of the workout is, in fact, anaerobic. The aerobic system is slower to turn on. It takes some minutes before the aerobic system has come in full operation.

In itself this workout is not ideal. When executed like this it has an aerobic interval workout, during which HR drops to 120/min in the recovery pauses (fig. 20).

Interpretation:

During a training method, the exertion phase should be longer than 3 min in blocks, e.g. 3–5–8 min. The continuous method must take 20–60 min. The intensity of the continuous workout is right. During the exertion phase HR is between 150 and 160 beats per minute, so between L2 and L4.

Power Training Workout by a Professional Cyclist

Test data: Lactate 2 = HR 150
            Lactate 3 = HR 155
            Lactate 4 = HR 160

Maximum HR = 175

The record (fig. 21) reflects a powertaking workout on the bicycle (riding uphill or with a head wind in a high gear).

Duration of the exertion phases is between 1 and 5 min. Number of repetitions should be 4 to 10× at the most. HR goes up in peaks over 160.

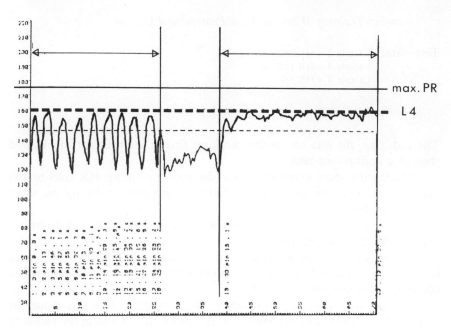

Fig. 20. See text.

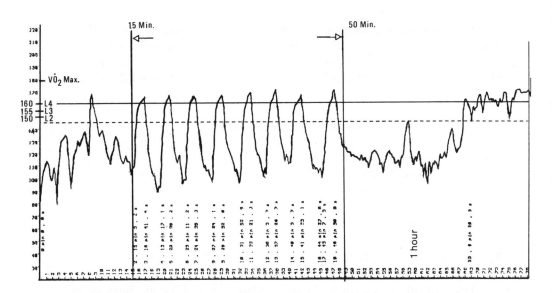

Fig. 21. See text.

Table 4 Pulse rate table for runners

PR/L 1	PR/L 2	PR/L 2.5	PR/L 3	PR/L 4	PR/L 1	PR/L 2	PR/L 2.5	PR/L 3	PR/L 4
149	162	164	167	171	122	132	134	137	140
149	163	165	168	172	122	133	135	138	141
150	164	166	169	173	123	134	136	139	142
151	164	167	170	174	124	135	137	140	143
152	165	168	171	175	125	136	138	141	144
153	166	169	172	176	126	137	139	142	145
154	167	170	173	177	127	138	140	142	146
155	168	171	174	178	128	139	141	143	147
156	169	172	175	179	129	140	142	144	148
156	170	173	176	180	129	141	143	145	149
157	171	174	177	181	130	142	144	146	150
158	172	175	178	182	131	143	145	147	151
159	173	176	179	183	132	144	146	148	152
160	174	177	180	184	133	145	147	149	153
161	175	178	181	185	134	146	148	150	154
162	176	179	182	186	135	147	149	151	155
163	177	180	183	187	136	147	150	152	156
163	178	180	183	188	136	148	151	153	157
164	179	181	184	189	137	149	152	154	158
165	180	182	185	190	138	150	153	155	159
166	181	183	186	191	139	151	154	156	160
167	181	184	187	192	140	152	155	157	161
168	182	185	188	193	141	153	156	158	162
169	183	186	189	194	142	154	156	159	163
170	184	187	190	195	142	155	157	160	164
170	185	188	191	196	143	156	158	161	165
171	186	189	192	197	144	157	159	162	166
172	187	190	193	198	145	158	160	163	167
173	188	191	194	199	146	159	161	164	168
174	189	192	195	200	147	160	162	165	169
					148	161	163	166	170

Interpretation:

This training workout is well executed. Note that the recovery following training is good (HR quickly drops to 90).

Heart Rate Lactate Table for Runners
There is a fixed relation between HR at the deflection point and the other training intensities.

Once the individual deflection HR is known, the other training intensities can be found with the help of the heart rate table for runners (table 4).

Various Training Forms and Races Related to the Heart
Rate Lactate Table for Runners
See figures 22–39 for details.

Training Workout of a 17-Year-Old Sprinter
Three series are run: 5×50 m, 5×60 m and 5×70 m.

Lactate after warm-up: 4.3 mmol/l.
Lactate after 3 min cool-down run: 2.9 mmol/l (starting lactate) (fig. 40).

First series	HR		HR	Time s	recovery min	lactate mmol/l
				Lactate at start 2.9		
1st 50m	110					
>	147	5.8	2	3.72nd 50m 132		
>	168	5.9	2	6.3		
3rd 50m	136	>	169	5.9	2	12.8
4th 50m	145	>	179	6.0	2	11.2
5th 50m	145	>	178	6.0	2	10.2

After this series a cool-down run of 10 min was completed.

Second series	HR		HR	Time s	recovery min	lactate mmol/l
				Lactate at start 7.1		
1st 60m	140	>	172	6.8	2	8.6
2nd 60m	150	>	179	7.0	2	11.1
3rd 60m	151	>	180	7.3	2	12.6
4th 60m	145	>	176	6.9	2	13.5
5th 60m	157	>	180	6.9	2	12.7

After this series a cool-down run of 12 min was completed.

Third series					Lactate at start 2.9	
	HR		HR	Time s	recovery min	lactate mmol/l
1st 70m	132	>	174	8.2	2	10.6
2nd 70m	154	>	181	8.0	2	15.5
3rd 70m	151	>	180	8.3	2	16.1
4th 70m	161	>	181	8.4	2	16.2
5th 70m	156	>	181	8.4	2	14.8

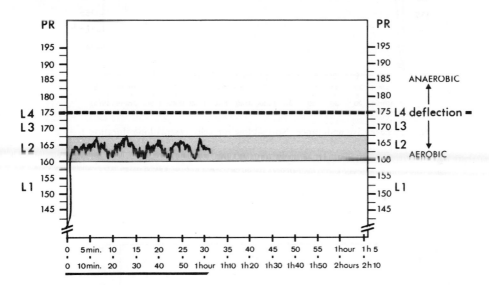

Fig. 22. Extensive endurance. Normal/intermediate intensity long duration L ± 1.5–2.5.

Interpretation:

This young sprinter trained three to four times a week in this way. During the last year there has been no improvement and the number of injuries has gone up. This workout has very high lactate values; it is to be considered as a very intensive lactate tolerance training method. As a sprint workout it is a complete failure. One such intense workout per week is likely sufficient; three to four must cause problems. This may explain both the lack of improvement and the increased incidence of injuries.

During sprint workouts lactate concentration must not go up so high. In order to avoid this recovery time must be longer. During this recovery time creatine phosphate (CP) and ATP (the phosphate battery) should be regenerated. It is striking how high HR is at the start of the sprints.

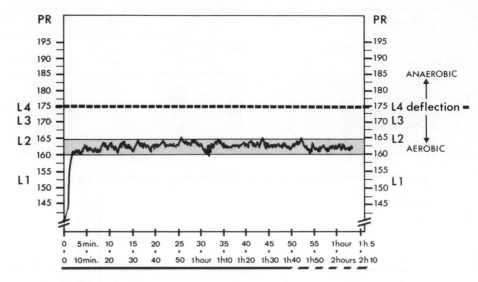

Fig. 23. Extensive endurance, Normal/low intensity (extra) long duration L 1–2.

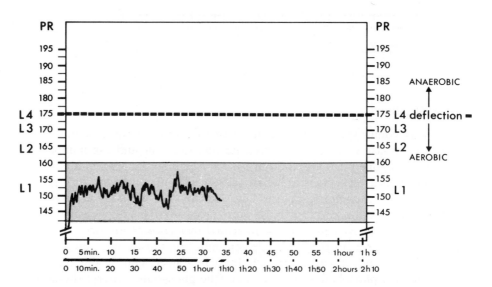

Fig. 24. Recovery workout (jog) low intensity short duration L 0.5–1.5.

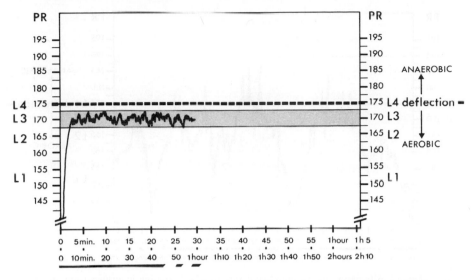

Fig. 25. Intensive endurance also test run 'high' intensity long/intermediate duration L 2.5–3.5.

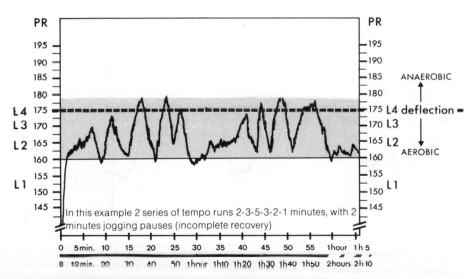

Fig. 26. Alternating pace method (structured) 'high' intensity, short to intermediate duration (may partially be tolerance workout) L 2.5–L 5.

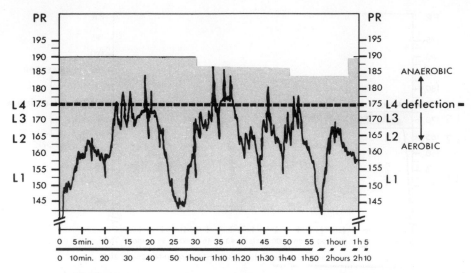

Fig. 27. Alternating pace method (not structured) alternating intensities (may be from very low to very high, from recovery to tolerance) L 0.5–L 10.

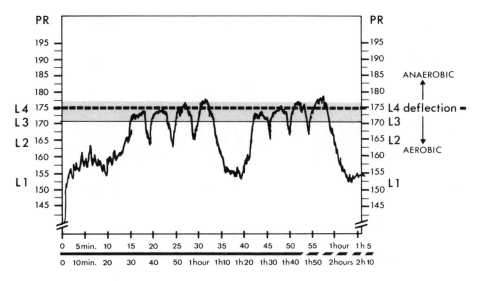

Fig. 28. Extensive intermediate intervals intermediate to high intensity 1–5 min L 3–L 4.5 with incomplete recovery.

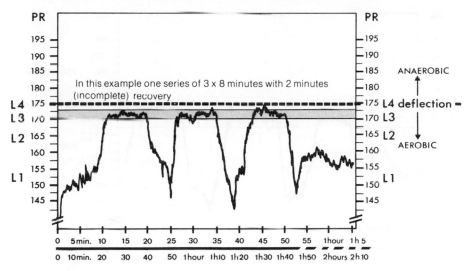

Fig. 29. Extensive long intervals intermediate to high intensity 5–15 min L 3–L 3.5 with incomplete recovery.

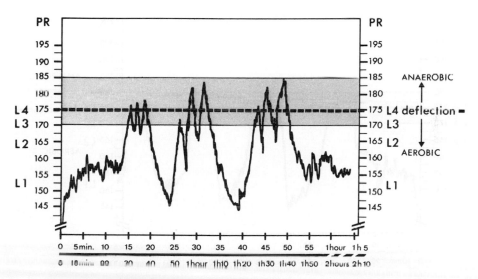

Fig. 30. Intense intervals high intensity (may be tolerance short duration, e.g. 1–1.5 min L 3–7 with incomplete recovery.

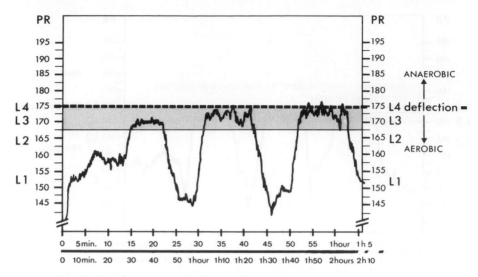

Fig. 31. Repetitions, extensive intermediate to high intensity long duration (e.g. 5– 15 min L 2.5–4 characteristic: complete recovery between runs.

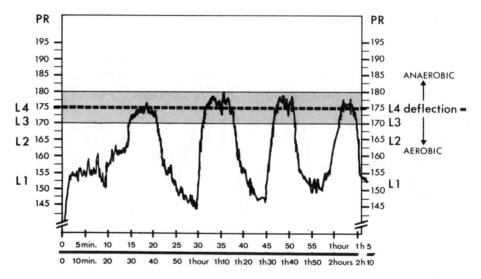

Fig. 32. Repetitions, intense high intensity (may be tolerance) intermediate duration (3– 5 min) L 3–5 with 'complete' recovery.

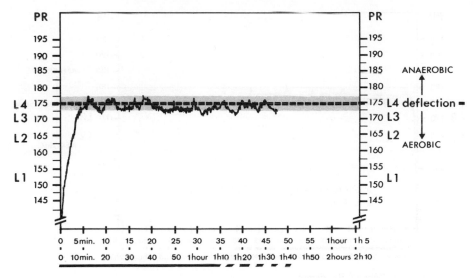

Fig. 33. Tolerence workout or race (e.g. race or test) length $\frac{1}{2}$ marathon intermediate to long duration high intensity L 3.5–5 intensity area: permanently around deflection L 4.

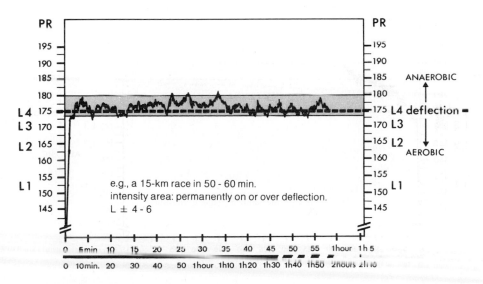

Fig. 34. Race of somewhat less than 1 h.

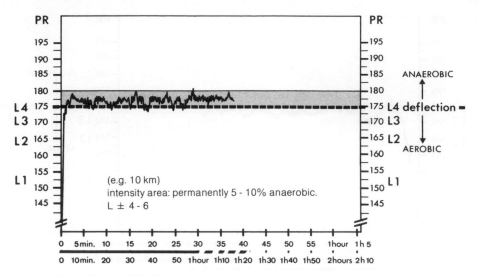

Fig. 35. Race of 30–40 min.

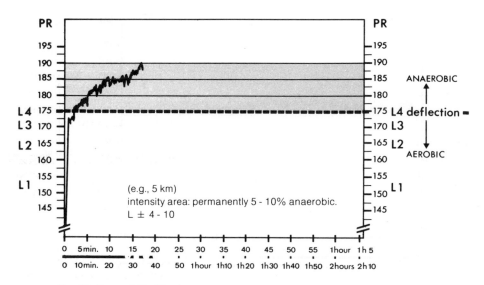

Fig. 36. Race of 15–20 min.

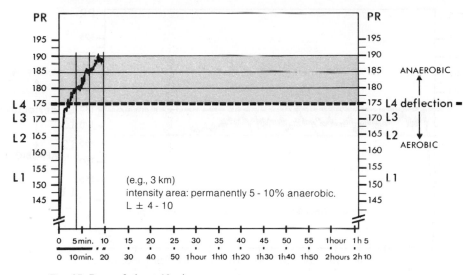

Fig. 37. Race of about 10 min.

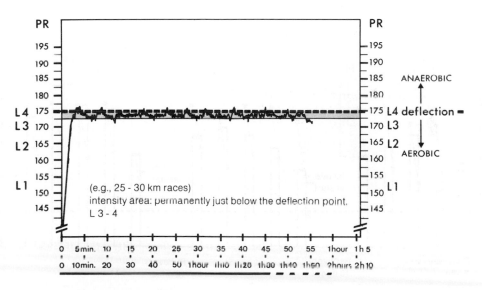

Fig. 38. Race of about 1.5–2 h.

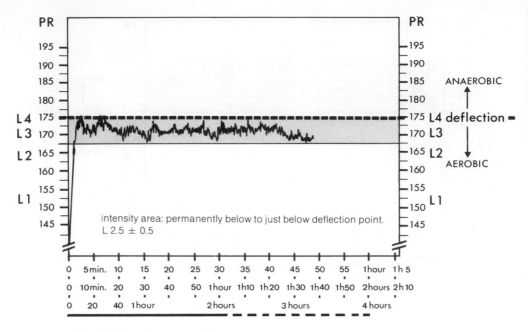

Fig. 39. Marathon, race of 2.5–3.5 h.

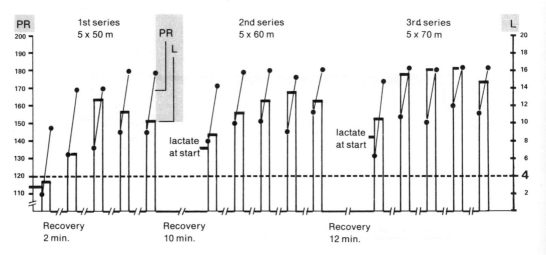

Fig. 40. See text.

Two Records of a Marathon Runner
(a) Eindhoven Marathon, October 1986 (fig. 41).
From the start to the 25th kilometer HR is over 165 beats per minute.
So this runner can perform 1 h and 48 min over his deflection point. Then
he cannot keep up his pace any longer. Running speed goes down rapidly.
So does his HR. The first 20 km split is covered in 1.23.27 and the second
in 1.54.42. Total time marathon: 3 h 27 min 28 s.

Interpretation:

A classic example of a failed marathon. On the basis of test data
training was adapted (test April) and the correct race intensity was
determined (test September).

April 1987	September 1987
Lactate 2 = HR 155	Lactate 2 = HR 156
Lactate 3 = HR 160	Lactate 3 = HR 161
Lactate 4 = HR 165	Lactate 4 = HR 165
V2 = 3.64 m/s	V2 = 4.00 m/s
V3 = 3.78 m/s	V3 = 4.10 m/s
V4 = 3.95 m/s	V4 = 4.19 m/s
V2.5 = 3 h 9 min	V2.5 = 2 h 53 min

These test data show that HR levels have not changed between April
and September, whereas his performance capacity has strongly increased.
The marathon time calculated with a running pace at lactate 2.5 mmol/l
(V2.5) has improved from 3 h 9 min to 2 h 53 min.
(b) Helmond Marathon, October 1987 (fig. 42).
A prudent start. He kept his HR at the beginning of the race
constantly under 160. Later in the race HR between 160 and 165, from 2
HR between 165 and 170.

1st 20 km split 1.24.21.
2nd 20 km split 1.23.01 (a so-called positive split).
Total time marathon 2 h 51 min 12.7 s.

Personal best. For the first time he ran under 3 h. At the beginning of
the race he kept himself under control.

Interpretation: well controlled, good marathon race.

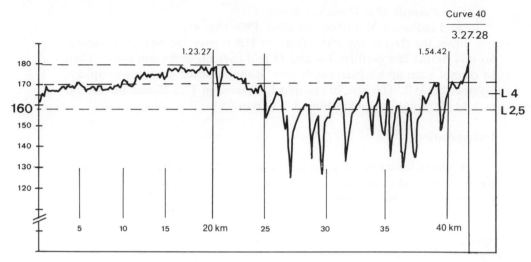

Fig. 41. See text.

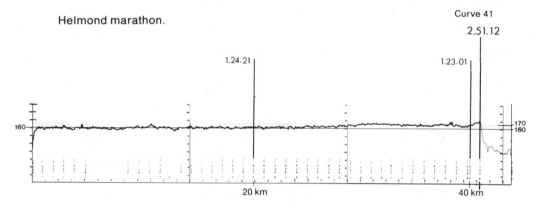

Fig. 42. See text.

Effect of Recent Bronchitis on Exercise Heart Rate in a Marathon Runner

Test data: Lactate 2 = HR 155
Lactate 3 = HR 160
Lactate 4 = HR 163

Maximum HR = 180 (fig. 43).

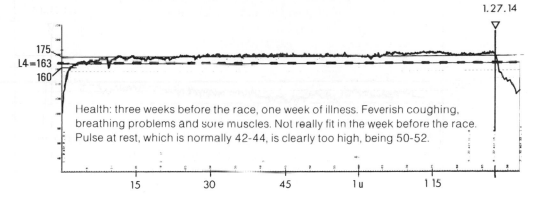

1.27.14

175
L4 = 163
160

Health: three weeks before the race, one week of illness. Feverish coughing, breathing problems and sore muscles. Not really fit in the week before the race. Pulse at rest, which is normally 42-44, is clearly too high, being 50-52.

15   30   45   1 u   1 15

Fig. 43. Half marathon Deurne, September 1987.

Race: did not run very well. Very high HR at relative low pace, HR being 175. Time 1.27.14. Poor recovery after race.

Interpretation.

Performance capacity clearly goes down when insufficiently recovered after an infectious disease. When doing exercise, HR goes up higher than normal values at relatively low speed (fig. 44).

Conditioning has strongly increased. It only makes sense to train or race when recovery after infectious disease is complete. An exertion as shown in figure 43 is no good at all. It would have been better not to run the race and take a good rest instead or do a light training workout at the most.

Soccer Training

Task: Run 6× uphill at maximum pace. When HR has gone down to 120 beats per minute make another start. During this form of training maximum lactate values are reached between 15 and 24 mmol/l. The high lactate values require a recovery period of at least 48 h. In this period the risk of injury is enormous. Training technical skills cannot be done well because co-ordination is disturbed in this recovery period.

This kind of training workouts often occur in soccer. The result is a decrease of endurance capacity. For these reasons this kind of workout during the preparatory phase should be avoided (fig. 45).

Soccer Match

In order to establish whether a soccer player performs intensely in a match measurements of heart rate and lactate concentration were made

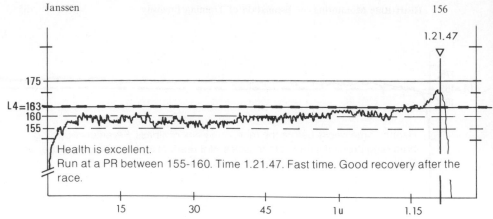

Fig. 44. Half marathon Eersel, February 1988.

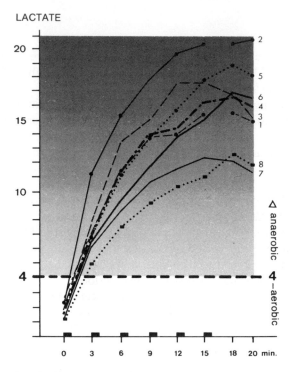

Fig. 45. Lactate curves of 8 soccer players during a workout in the preparatory phase to the new season [18].

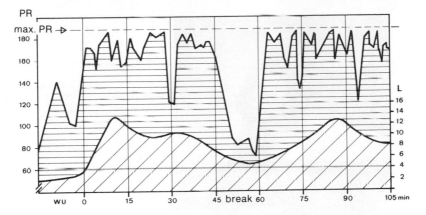

Fig. 46. Pulse rate and blood lactate of a center player during a soccer match in the Swedish first division.

(fig. 46). Apparently top soccer players have heart rates over 85% of their maximum and lactate of >8 mmol/l during a large part of the match.

For professional soccer players the average oxygen intake in a normal match turns out to be almost 80% of the $\dot{V}O_2$ max. This means that a soccer player should have an excellent aerobic endurance capacity and a soccer specific anaerobic endurance capacity.

The exertion in a soccer match often has an anaerobic character with all the nasty consequences of it, such as disturbed co-ordination and an enhanced risk of injury.

Conclusion

HR registrations of races and training workouts supply an objective picture of the exercise. For this reason alone it makes sense to register HR regularly. From analyses of HR records it appears that many mistakes are made during workouts and races. It is often difficult to estimate the right intensity of the exercise, resulting for instance in lactate tolerance training when endurance training was intended. HR records provide an excellent means to avoid these mistakes and to teach the athlete the correct subjective feeling for a given intensity. HR registration equipment may be used to guide training directly; but the biggest advantage is that the athlete gains an insight into the manner in which he trains. This enables him to have optimal benefits of his training by which performance level may rise.

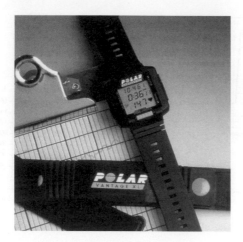

Fig. 47. For explanation see text.

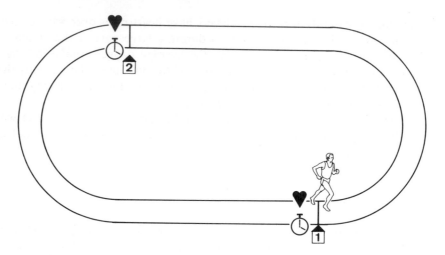

Fig. 48. For explanation see text.

References

1 Israel S, Weber W: Probleme der langzeit Ausdauer im Sport. Leipzig, Barth, 1972.
2 Jablonski D, Liesen H, Kraus I, Mödder H: Intensitätssteuerung und Leistungs-
beurteilung beim Jogging. Beziehung zwischen Atemschrittfrequenz und Blutlaktat-
spiegel. Fortschr Med 1985;4:47–50.
3 Astrand PO: Textbook of Work Physiology. New York, McGraw-Hill, 1986, pp
405–410.

4 van den Bosch J: De test van Conconi in de praktijk.
5 Conconi C: Determination of the anaerobic threshold by non-invasive field test in runners. J Appl Physiol 1982;52:869–873.
6 Claes J: Een evalutie van BF bepalingen. Sportmed Tijd 1984;2045–2061.
7 Karvonen J, Vuorimaa T: Heart rate and exercise intensity during sports activities. Practical application. Sports Med 1988;5:303–312.
8 Karvonen K, Kubica R, Wilk B, Wnorowski J, Krasicki S, Kalli S: Effects of skating and diagonal skiing techniques on results and some physiological variables. Can J Sport Sci 1989;14:117–121.
9 Heck H, Mader A, Hess G, Mücke S, Müller R, Hollmann W: Justification of the 4-mmol/l lactate threshold. Int J Sports Med 1985;6:117–130.
10 Liesen H: Trainingssteuerung im Hochleistungssport: einige Aspekte und Beispiele. Dtsch Z Sportmed 1985;12:8–18.
11 Probst H: Praktische Durchführung des Conconitests. Leichtathletiek 1988;6:184–186.
12 Janssen PGJM: Training, Lactate, Pulse Rate. Oulu, Liitto Oy, 1989, pp 42–101.
13 Binkhorst RA: Anaerobic drempel. Gen Sport 1981;3:78–79.
14 Hollmann W: Historical remarks on the development of the aerobic-anaerobic threshold up to 1966. Int J Sports Med 1985;6:109–116.
15 Hollmann W: Die aerobe Leistungsfähigkeit. Aspekte von Gesundheit und Sport. Spektrum Wissenschaft 1986:48–58.
16 Rispens P, Lamberts R: Physiological, Biomechanical and Technical Aspects of Speed Skating. Groningen, University of Groningen, 1985.
17 Stegmann D: Bestimmung der individuellen Schwelle bei unterschiedlich Ausdauertrainierten auf Grund des Verhaltens der Laktatkinetik während der Arbeits- und Erholungsphase. Dtsch Z Sportmed 1981;8:213–220.
18 Karvonen J, Chwalbinska-Moneta J, Pekkarinen H, Kangas J: Die Belastungsintensität während Lauf- und Rollerskitraining bei Skilangläufern. Schweiz Z Sportmed 1982;30:101–105.
19 Mader A: Umfang und Intensität im Dauerlauftraining von Mittelstreckenläuferinen der DLV und Massnahmen zur individuellen Trainings- und Wettkampfoptimierung.
20 Hollmann W: Sportmedizin Arbeits- und Trainingsgrundlagen. Stuttgart, Schattauer, 1980.
21 Nonella L: Feldtest zur Ermittlung der anaeroben Schwelle. Läufer 1986.
22 Mader A: Evaluation of lactic acid anaerobic energy contribution by determination of postexercise lactic acid concentration of ear capillary blood in middle distance runners and swimmers. Exerc Physiol 1978;4:187–200.
23 Mellerowicz H: Training. Tijdstroom, 1977.
24 Olbrecht J: De praktische betekenis van laktaatonderzoekingen voor trainigsplanning en trainingsuitvoering. Lezing te Diepenbeek op 10.11.1984. Sportmed Tijd 1985.
25 von Wanner HU: Subjektive Einstufung der Belastung bei Ausdauerleistungen. Dtsch Z Sportmed 1985;4:102–112.

Peter G.J.M. Janssen, MD, Deltasingel 29, NL-5751SL Deurne (The Netherlands)

Karvonen J, Lemon PWR, Iliev I (eds): Medicine in Sports Training and Coaching.
Med Sport Sci. Basel, Karger, 1992, vol 35, pp 160–173

Nutritional Factors in Strength and Endurance Training

Peter W.R. Lemon

School of Biomedical Sciences and Department of Physical Education,
Kent State University, Kent, Ohio, USA

Contents

Introduction

Despite the fact that nutrition can play a critical role in exercise performance [1] few coaches or athletes are well trained in nutritional science. This inadequate training combined with an intense desire to excel frequently leads to bizarre nutritional practices in athletes. Apparently, looking for a possible advantage or simply duplicating procedures that they believe competitors are using, many athletes self-experiment with extremely vast quantities of particular nutrients. It is routinely assumed that if a small amount is (or may be) good, a large amount must be better. Such practices frequently have little scientific basis and can be extremely costly not only because many of the products consumed are expensive but also because some are hazardous to one's health [2].

Although there are many theoretical beneficial effects of nutritional supplementation on exercise performance, in most cases there is little or no objective data indicating that a desired effect actually occurs. Clearly, this is one area of the preparation for athletic competition that requires much more study. For these reasons and because some nutritional manipulations can safely enhance exercise performance, it is essential that both coaches and athletes become more knowledgeable about nutrition. The purpose of this paper is to review several of the more important nutritional factors known to influence either strength or endurance performance. These include intake of energy, macronutrients (carbohydrate, fat, and protein), and water/electrolytes. Other interesting areas of nutrition for athletes (such as vitamins and minerals) have been reviewed recently [3, 4] and will not be repeated here.

Energy

Adequate energy intake is critical for all individuals but especially for athletes because maintenance of body mass depends upon the energy balance equation (energy intake = energy output). When energy (food) intake exceeds output (exercise), body mass is increased. Conversely when energy output exceeds input, body mass is decreased. The sensitivity of the equation is such that even a small daily imbalance can lead to substantial changes in body mass over time. For example over one year, if intake is 200 (~ 840 kJ/ day) kcal/day (about 3 slices of bread) more than output the resulting gain in mass would be about 10 kg (200 kcal/day × 365 days/year/7,700 kcal/kg). This gain in mass could be largely muscle for a body builder engaged in regular strength training or largely fat for his/her more sedentary counterpart.

Daily energy requirement is usually expressed per kg body mass because the most important factor influencing it is basal metabolic rate, which is largely determined by body mass. Although estimates of energy requirements based on large numbers of essentially sedentary subjects are available [5, 6], requirements for those engaged in regular exercise training are at least 40–85% greater (table 1). The need for increased energy intake is readily apparent for endurance athletes because of the large expenditures involved in their prolonged training sessions. However, several investigations [8–10] indicate that the energy requirement of strength athletes may be elevated to a similar extent. Unlike endurance athletes, the increased energy requirement for strength athletes is probably not related to excessive exercise expenditures during training [11] because the actual time for muscular contraction for these athletes is relatively brief (a large percentage of each training session is taken by rest/recovery). Rather, the elevated energy requirement may be caused by an increased basal metabolic rate required by the enlarged muscle mass of these athletes.

Table 1. Mean daily energy expenditure for men [modified from ref. 7]

Group	Daily energy expenditure		
	kJ · kg^{-1}	kcal · kg^{-1}	%
Nonathletes	205	49	100
Cross-country skiers	377	90	184
Marathon runners	364	87	178
Weightlifters	318	76	155
Shotput, discus throwers	285	68	139

Table 2. Approximate whole body carbohydrate stores for a 70-kg individual [15]

Site	Carbohydrate store g
Muscle	300–600
Liver	0–90
Extracellular fluid	8–11

For both strength and endurance athletes the energy balance equation must remain positive or losses in muscle mass and strength will result. To reduce the chances of losing body mass it is recommended that athletes increase the number of daily meals to 5 or 6. In addition, when expenditures are very high it may not be possible to consume adequate quantities of solid food because of its excessive bulk. Therefore, in addition to large quantities of solid food many athletes could benefit from the use of nutritional beverages high in energy [12–14].

Carbohydrate

Carbohydrate (CHO) is stored in the body in two forms: as glucose in extracellular water (primarily in the blood) and as glycogen (a long chain of glucose molecules) in muscle and liver (table 2). It is a critical nutrient in the athlete's diet not only because it is the major fuel that provides energy during intense exercise but also because the body's supply is relatively small. In fact, it is possible to significantly deplete CHO stores during one exercise bout (1–3 h continuous exercise at moderate pace [16] or 5–15 min of intense intermittent exercise [17]). This means that both strength and endurance athletes may routinely exhaust their CHO stores during either training or competition. When this occurs several effects result. First, alternative energy sources must be used acutely which would adversely affect performance because they necessitate a slower exercise pace. Second, the potential exists for chronically reduced CHO availability leading to compromised training sessions.

It is now well established that body CHO stores can be increased substantially by appropriate dietary practices [18–20]. To minimize the chances of having insufficient CHO available it is necessary to have large quantities of CHO (8–10 g/kg body weight) in the diet of both strength and endurance athletes. Although many athletes realize the advantages of high CHO diets, few athletes consume this much CHO. In order to do so, one must consider both the type of CHO and the timing of its ingestion.

First, CHO are classified according to their ability to increase blood glucose (glycemic index). Although not well studied, it appears that high and moderate glycemic foods produce greater rates of CHO storage. As a result, an athlete should be sure to consume the majority of CHO in these forms. Examples of foods with a high or moderate glycemic index include: bread, chocolate, rice, whole wheat cereal, oatmeal, pasta, potatoes, corn, bananas, raisins, oranges, grapes, sugar, honey, and sports drinks. Examples of low glycemic foods include: apples, cherries, dates, figs, grapefruit, peaches, plums, beans, peas, fructose, and dairy products. Second, in order to maximize CHO availability athletes must consume large amounts of CHO before, during, and following exercise. In general, ∼0.7–0.8 g/kg of CHO every 2 h maximizes CHO storage [21, 22], so multiple small meals are probably best. Although such a schedule would provide sufficient CHO over 24 h, practically it is not possible to eat every 2 h, especially during sleep. Therefore, when frequent meals are not possible athletes must consume enough CHO in the previous meal to cover the period of time until the next meal. This means that most athletes will consume several large meals and many small meals (snacks) throughout each 24-hour period.

Post-Exercise Period

Immediately following exercise (∼2 h), the rate of glycogen storage is higher than at any other time [22] and, therefore, this is probably the single most critical time to ingest CHO (Fig. 1). Unfortunately, athletes are rarely hungry at this time and it may be difficult to get them to consume sufficient CHO during this critical period unless high CHO sport drinks and/or foods (candy bars, raisins, bananas, etc.) are readily available.

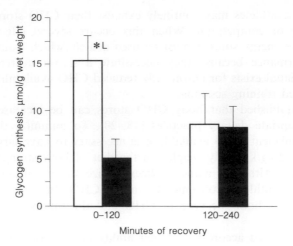

Fig. 1. Muscle glycogen storage during the first and second 2 h after 70 min of glycogen-depleting exercise when CHO (2 g/kg body weight of a 25% CHO solution) was ingested immediately (open bars) or 2 hours after the exercise (filled bars).*L = Significantly (p < 0.05) greater than both the 0- to 120-min time period without CHO ingestion (basal rate) and the 120- to 240-min period when CHO ingestion occurred during the second 2 h [22].

Pre-Exercise Period

During the week preceding an event where CHO stores might be limiting, it is possible to substantially increase the body's CHO stores by minor manipulations of both diet and training practices [23]. This involves consuming a moderate CHO intake (~ 5 g/kg · d^{-1}) 4–7 days before the event followed by a high CHO intake (~ 8–10 g/kg · d^{-1}) for 3 days immediately prior to the event. In addition, training should be reduced (by about 50%) 5 days before and again 3 days before the event. Finally, the day prior to the event should be a rest day. If training is not reduced, the additional CHO in the diet will not be stored as it will be needed for fuel during training. Further, it is important to understand that such a modest reduction in training the week before a competition will have no detrimental effect on exercise capacity.

On the day of the event, there is accumulating evidence [24] that intake of 200–250 g of high glycemic index CHO that is low in fat and fiber approximately 4 h prior to the event will enhance performance in events where CHO stores are limiting.

During Event Period

For prolonged exercise (>2 h) where athletes fatigue due to CHO depletion, high glyccmic CHO intake throughout the exercise bout can enable an athlete to continue for an additional 30–60 min [19]. The ingested CHO does not seem to affect muscle glycogen use but rather maintains blood glucose concentration which appears to provide a greater percentage of the energy when exercise is prolonged (fig. 2). Although ingestion of very large amounts of CHO (~200 g) near the point of fatigue may enable an athlete to continue, it is far superior to consume smaller amounts (30–60 g/h) at regular intervals during prolonged exercise. Glucose polymers (maltodextrins), which arc chains of 7–13 glucose units produced by hydrolysis of starch, found in many sport drinks are an excellent CHO source because they have less bulk and as a result are more easily ingested and absorbed than many solid CHO [12–14, 25]. Intake of CHO during lower intensity exercise or rest recovery periods of intermittent type exercise is also beneficial [12, 26–28]. This may be due to a reduced use of stored CHO or perhaps a greater rate of storage. Finally, it should be remembered that CHO intake during activities that are not limited by CHO stores (low intensity exercise or very brief intense efforts) provides no advantage during competition, although diets high in CHO are clearly required to support the more prolonged training sessions necessary for successful performances in these activities. Examples of this type of situation include many of the strength/power sports.

Protein

Protein is necessary for life. It is found throughout the body but primarily in skeletal muscle. There are many different proteins each made up of a unique mixture of amino acids. Although our bodies have the ability to make protein from amino acids they arc only able to produce some of the necessary amino acids. The others are called essential (indispensable) amino acids (table 3) because they must be obtained via the diet. If these are not consumed in adequate quantities and in the same meal, the body's ability to produce protein is impaired. Over time, this leads to decreases in muscle mass and strength. Unfortunately, only some foods (dairy products, eggs, fish, meat, poultry) or food combinations (corn/rice plus beans, corn plus peas, lentils plus bread, etc) contain all these amino acids. This means that the athlete must be careful to not only consume enough total protein but also the right combinations of foods to insure an adequate mixture of the essential amino acids is available for protein synthesis. This is especially true for athletes following strictly vegetarian diets.

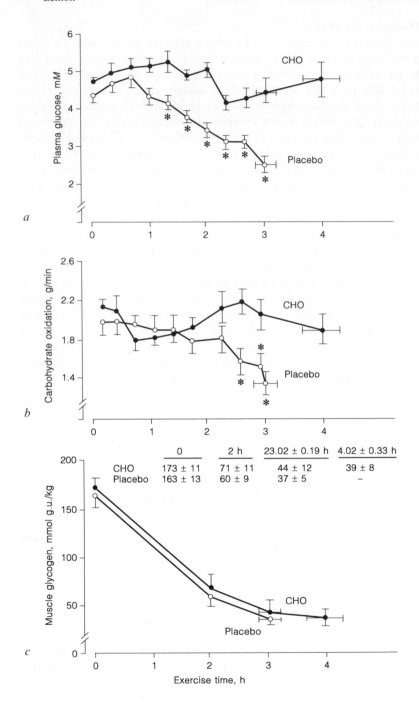

	0	2 h	23.02 ± 0.19 h	4.02 ± 0.33 h
CHO	173 ± 11	71 ± 11	44 ± 12	39 ± 8
Placebo	163 ± 13	60 ± 9	37 ± 5	–

Table 3. Essential or indispensable amino acids

Histidine
Isoleucine
Leucine
Lysine
Methionine/cysteine
Phenylalanine/tyrosine
Threonine
Tryptophan
Valine

In general, during and immediately after exercise protein production decreases and protein breakdown increases. Then at some point, protein production increases again and exceeds protein breakdown. However, the magnitude and time course of these effects differ between endurance and strength exercise [29]. As a result, regular training with one or the other type of exercise produces vastly different body types. With endurance exercise, protein is necessary to increase mitochondrial (enzymatic) protein and as an auxiliary exercise fuel [30]. In contrast, with strength exercise protein is needed so it is possible to increase muscle mass (myofibrillar protein) and strength [31].

Considerable controversy has existed for years between coaches/athletes and nutritionists regarding whether or not regular training alters protein requirements [32–35]. At least part of the confusion is due to technical problems with many of the experiments designed to answer this question. These include methodological difficulties and inadequate control of one or more of several factors (diet composition, energy intake, exercise intensity, exercise duration, training status, environment, gender, and age) now known to affect protein metabolism. Although definitive recommendations must await further study, the weight of current evidence suggests that dietary protein requirements of athletes exceed those of the general population. It appears that strength athletes should consume ~ 1.2–1.7 g protein/ kg $\cdot$ d^{-1} (beginners toward the high end [36]; experienced strength athletes

---

Fig. 2. Plasma glucose (*a*), CHO oxidation (*b*) and muscle glycogen concentration (*c*) during exercise with ingestion of either CHO (2 g/kg body weight of a 50% CHO solution ●) or placebo (○) every 20 min. *Placebo significantly ($p < 0.05$) lower than CHO [19].

toward the low end [37]) and endurance athletes $\sim 1.2-1.4$ g/kg $\cdot$ d^{-1} [35]. This represents increases of $\sim 50-112\%$ relative to current recommendations [5, 6]. However, it may not be necessary to increase the protein intake of many athletes because as a result of very high energy intakes they may already be consuming this quantity of protein, i.e. an energy intake of 5,000 kcal ($\sim 21{,}000$ kJ) with only 10% protein would contain 125 g protein (~ 1.9 g/kg $\cdot$ d^{-1} for a 70-kg athlete). Therefore, it is necessary to carefully assess one's diet and exercise habits before it can be determined whether supplemental dietary protein will enhance athletic performance.

Fat

Fat is the major energy reserve in the body. It is found primarily in adipose tissue but also in muscle. In terms of potential energy, the body's store of fat is extremely vast. To illustrate, a male endurance athlete weighing 60 kg would have ~ 6 kg of fat (assuming 10% of his body weight is fat). This fat could provide the sole source of energy for this athlete to run continuously at a moderate pace for several days. Clearly, even for this lean athlete fat stores are not limiting for exercise. However, for fat to be utilized it must first be broken down into its component parts (glycerol and free fatty acids) in the fat cell. Via the blood, glycerol travels to the liver where it is used to produce glucose and the free fatty acids are transported to other tissues, especially muscle, where they can be used for exercise energy. Fatty acids require more oxygen than CHO and, therefore, cannot be used during very high intensity exercise. However, they provide a significant percentage of exercise energy during low and moderate intensity exercise and also during the later stages of prolonged exercise when CHO stores are becoming exhausted. Unfortunately, because oxygen supply to muscle is limiting and free fatty acids require more oxygen to provide comparable energy the increased contribution from fat means that one's exercise pace must be reduced.

Interestingly, as one becomes endurance trained it is possible to use fat for energy at greater exercise intensities [38]. This new ability is the result of changes in both free fatty acid delivery and utilization and has a significant effect on endurance performance because its use conserves the athletes' limited CHO stores.

Intake of some fat is necessary to obtain several essential nutrients. However, most individuals consume more fat than they need. This should be avoided as diets high in fat are associated with cardiovascular disease [39]. Fat intake should be no greater than 30% of energy intake and supplemental fat intake is not necessary for training or competition.

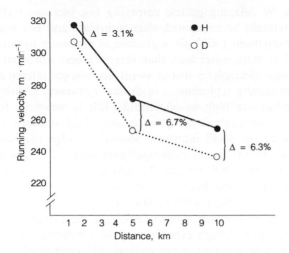

Fig. 3. Effect of dehydration on endurance running performance. H = Hydrated; D = dehydrated. Observed times were significantly (p < 0.05) faster for the hydrated runners during both 5- and 10-km races [40].

Water and Electrolytes

Water is the largest and perhaps the most important single component of the body (50–70% of body mass). It is possible to survive for several weeks without food but for only a few days without water. During exercise, depending on the intensity and duration, as well as environment and prior training, large losses of body water (> 2 litres/h) can occur due to sweating. The resulting dehydration not only reduces the athlete's capacity to perform (fig. 3) but can lead to serious medical complications and even death. For obvious reasons, it is essential to do everything possible to minimize the chances of dehydration [41]. Important precautions include: wearing appropriate clothing (light colored, porous material); avoiding hottest times of the day; acclimatizing slowly over 1–2 weeks; and most importantly consuming adequate fluids before, during, and after exercise.

Composition and Volume of Ingested Fluids

Clearly, it is critical to replace water losses due to sweating. However, it is possible and advantageous to provide exercise fuel (CHO) at the same time. Generally, high CHO solutions (150–200 g glucose polymers/liter) reduce fluid availability by delaying gastric emptying but increase CHO delivery and, therefore, should be consumed when substrate and not fluid is limiting. Lower CHO solutions ($<20-30$ g glucose or glucose polymers/liter) deliver less CHO but more water and, therefore, are best when fluid, not CHO, is limiting. Most electrolytes lost in sweat are not considered to be substantial enough to require replacement in drinks. However, addition of sodium chloride (perhaps as high as 60 mmol/l [42]) is beneficial for several reasons. First, it increases both glucose and fluid delivery by stimulating their uptake in the small intestine. Second, it helps maintain extracellular fluid volume. Third, in very prolonged exercise (>4 h) it helps prevent hyponatremia (a rare but potentially serious situation where sodium concentration in the blood becomes too low [43, 44]). Frequent ingestion of small volumes of fluid ($100-200$ ml/$15-20$ min) is recommended because the resulting stomach volumes increase fluid delivery by stimulating gastric emptying. Although experimental data indicate that the temperature of the fluid to be ingested is not critical [45], cool drinks are recommended because the athletes are more likely to drink them. Post exercise fluid replacement should follow the same principles with the total volume consumed determined by changes in body weight. Intake of $400-500$ ml of fluid $15-20$ min prior to the event may also help.

Conclusion

Although it is frequently stated that nutrition plays a critical role in an athlete's performance, relatively little is known about many nutritional manipulations used routinely by athletes. Further, a great deal of misinformation exists. It is clear that the nutrient needs of strength/endurance athletes are different than the general population. For example, the requirements for energy, CHO, protein, water, and some electrolytes (especially sodium) are greater for athletes. Actual requirements depend primarily on the event and the size of the athlete but other factors such as training status, environment, gender, and perhaps even age may also be important. Much more study is needed to provide objective data regarding the efficacy/safety of many of the nutritional practices employed by today's athletes. It is strongly recommended that both coaches and athletes receive more training in nutritional science so they can better evaluate the specific nutritional fads that exist today as well as those that will undoubtedly arise in the future. Finally, none of the nutritional manipulations discussed should be utilized for the first time associated with a competitive event because individual tolerances vary. Be sure you know how you will respond by experimenting during training sessions.

References

1 Williams MH: Nutritional Aspects of Human Physical and Athletic Performance. Springfield, Thomas, 1985.
2 Teman AJ, Hainline B: Eosinophilia-myalgia syndrome. Phys Sportsmed 1991;19:81–86.
3 van der Beek EJ: Vitamin supplementation and physical exercise performance. J Sports Sci 1991;9:77–89.
4 Clarkson PM: Minerals: Exercise performance and supplementation in athletes. J Sports Sci 1991;9:91–116.
5 Food and Agricultural Organization, World Health Organization and United Nations University: Energy and Protein Requirements. World Health Organization Tech Rep Ser 724. Geneva, WHO, 1985.
6 US Food and Nutrition Board: Recommended Dietary Allowances, vol 10. Washington, National Academy of Sciences, 1989.
7 American College of Sports Medicine: Encyclopedia of Sports Medicine. New York, MacMillan, 1971, pp 1128–1129.
8 Celejowa I, Homa M: Food intake, nitrogen and energy balance in Polish weight lifters during a training camp. Nutr Metab 1970;12:259–274.
9 Dragan I, Vasiliu A, Georgescu E: Effects of increased supply of protein on elite weight lifters; in Galesloot TE, Tinbergen BJ (eds): Milk Proteins 84. Wageningen, The Netherlands, 1985, pp 99–103.
10 Laritcheva HA, Yolovaya NI, Shubin VI, Smirnow PV: Study of energy expenditure and protein needs of top weight lifters, in Pariakova J, Rogozkin VA (eds): Nutrition, Physical Fitness, and Health. Baltimore, University Park Press, 1978, pp 155–163.
11 Tarnopolsky MA, Atkinson SA, MacDougall JD, Senor BB, Lemon PWR, Schwarcz H: Whole body leucine metabolism during and after resistance exercise in fed humans. Med Sci Sports Exerc 1991;23:326–333.
12 Brouns F, Saris WHM, Stroecken J, Beckers E, Thijssen R, Rehrer NJ, ten Hoor F: Eating, drinking, and cycling. A controlled Tour de France simulation study, part 1. Int J Sports Med 1989;10(suppl 1):S32–S40.
13 Brouns F, Saris WHM, Stroecken J, Beckers E, Thijssen R, Rehrer NJ, ten Hoor F: Eating, drinking, and cycling. A controlled Tour de France simulation study, part 2. Int J Sports Med 1989;10(suppl 1):S41–S48.
14 Brouns F, Saris WHM, Beckers E, Adlercreutz H, van der Vusse GJ, Keizer HA, Kuipers H, Menheere P, Wangenmakers AJM, ten Hoor F: Metabolic changes induced by sustained exhaustive cycling and diet manipulation. Int J Sports Med 1989;10(suppl 1):S49–S62.
15 Saltin B, Gollnick PD: Fuel for muscular exercise: Role of carbohydrate; in Horton ES, Terjung RL (eds): Exercise, Nutrition and Energy Metabolism. New York, MacMillan, 1988, p 47.
16 Hermansen L, Hultman E, Saltin B: Muscle glycogen during prolonged severe exercise. Acta Physiol Scand 1967;71:129–139.
17 MacDougall JD, Ward GR, Sale DG, Sutton JR: Muscle glycogen repletion after high intensity exercise. J Appl Physiol 1977;42:129–132.
18 Costill DL: Carbohydrates for exercise: Dietary demands for optimal performance. Int J Sports Med 1988;9:1–18.
19 Coyle EF, Coggan AR, Hemmert MK, Ivy JL: Muscle glycogen utilization during prolonged strenuous exercise when fed carbohydrate. J Appl Physiol 1986;61:165–172.
20 Sherman WM: Carbohydrate feedings before and after exercise; in Lamb DR, Williams MH (eds): Perspectives in Exercise Science and Sports Medicine, vol 4. Ergogenics –

The Enhancement of Exercise and Sports Performance. Indianapolis, Benchmark Press, 1991, pp 1–34.

21   Blom PC, Hostmark AT, Vaage O, Vardal KR, Maehlum S: Effect of different post exercise sugar diets on the rate of muscle glycogen synthesis. Med Sci Sports Exerc 1987;19:491–496.

22   Ivy JL, Katz AL, Cutler CL, Sherman WM, Coyle EF: Muscle glycogen synthesis after exercise: Effect of time of carbohydrate ingestion. J Appl Physiol 1988;64:1480–1485.

23   Sherman WM, Costill DL, Fink WJ, Miller JM: The effect of exercise and diet manipulation on muscle glycogen and its subsequent use during performance. Int J Sports Med 1981;2:114–118.

24   Coyle EF: Timing and method of increased carbohydrate intake to cope with heavy training, competition and recovery. J Sports Sci 1991;9:29–52.

25   Rehrer NJ: Aspects of dehydration and rehydration during exercise; in Brouns F (ed): Advances in Nutrition and Top Sport. Med Sport Sci. Basel, Karger, 1991, vol 32, pp 128–146.

26   Muckle DS: Glucose syrup ingestion and team performance in soccer. Br J Sports Med 1973;7:340–343.

27   Simard C, Tremblay A, Jobin M: Effects of carbohydrate intake before and during an ice hockey match on blood and muscle energy substrates. Res Quart Exerc Sport 1988;59:144–147.

28   Kuipers H, Keizer HA, Brouns F, Saris WHM: Carbohydrate feedings and glycogen synthesis during exercise in man. Eur J Appl Physiol 1987;410:652–656.

29   Booth FW, Watson PA: Control of adaptations in protein levels in response to exercise. Fed Proc 1985;44:2293–2300.

30   Lemon PWR: Protein and exercise: Update 1987. Med Sci Sports Exerc 1987;9(5, suppl):S179–S190.

31   Lemon PWR: Protein and amino acid needs of the strength athlete. Int J Sports Nutr 1991;1:127–145.

32   von Liebig J: Animal Chemistry or Organic Chemistry in its Application to Physiology and Pathology (translated by Gregory G). London, Taylor & Walton, 1842.

33   Cathcart EP: Influence of muscle work on protein metabolism. Physiol Rev 1925;5:225–243.

34   Butterfield GE: Amino acids and high protein diets; in Lamb DR, Williams MH (eds): Perspectives in Exercise Science and Sports Medicine, vol 4. Ergogenics – The Enhancement of Exercise and Sport Performance. Indianapolis, Benchmark Press, 1991, pp 87–122.

35   Lemon PWR: Effect of exercise on protein requirements. J Sports Sci 1991;9:53–70.

36   Lemon PWR, MacDougall JD, Tarnopolsky MA, Atkinson SA: Effect of dietary protein and body building exercise on muscle mass and strength gains. Can J Sport Sci 1990;15(4):14S.

37   Tarnopolsky MA, MacDougall JD, Atkinson SA: Influence of protein intake and training status on nitrogen balance and lean body mass. J Appl Physiol 1988;64:187–193.

38   Bjorntorp P: Importance of fat as a support nutrient for energy: Metabolism of athletes. J Sports Sci 1991;9:71–76.

39   Castelli WP: Epidemiology of coronary heart disease. The Framingham study. Am J Med 1984;76:4–12.

40   Armstrong LE, Costill DL, Fink WJ: Influence of diuretic-induced dehydration on competitive running performance. Med Sci Sports Exerc 1985;17:456–461.

41   American College of Sports Medicine: Position stand on the prevention of thermal injuries during distance running. Med Sci Sports Exerc 1984;16:ix–xiv.

42   Maughan RJ: Fluid and electrolyte loss and replacement in exercise. J Sports Sci 1991;9:117–142.

43   Noakes TD, Goodwin N, Rayner BL, Branken T, Taylor RKN: Water intoxication: A possible complication during endurance exercise. Med Sci Sports Exerc 1985;17:370–375.

44   Noakes TD, Norman RJ, Buck RH, Godlonton J, Stevenson K, Pittaway D: The incidence of hyponatremia during prolonged ultraendurance exercise. Med Sci Sports Exerc 1990;22:165–170.

45   McArthur KE, Feldman M: Gastric acid secretion, gastrin release, and gastric temperature in humans as affected by liquid meal temperature. Am J Clin Nutr 1989;49:51–54.

Dr. P.W.R. Lemon, Applied Physiology Research Laboratory,
Kent State University, Kent, OH 44242 (USA)

Karvonen J, Lemon PWR, Iliev I (eds): Medicine in Sports Training and Coaching.
Med Sport Sci. Basel, Karger, 1992, vol 35, pp 174–188

Overtraining

Juha Karvonen

Department of Clinical Physiology, University Hospital of Tampere, Finland

Contents

Introduction

The relationship between performance gains and training load is nonlinear. As training exceeds some limit, results gradually start to deteriorate. This state is known as overtraining, and it is due to excessive exertion.

During overtraining, performance results achieved by an athlete fail to improve or even get worse despite vigorous conscientious training. In addition to decreased performance, various functional disturbances are typical of overtraining. Coaches should be familiar with this phenomenon because it can be prevented. However, to do so requires close monitoring of the athlete's training as well as the use of physiological and biochemical indicators of training load [1].

Reasons for Overtraining

According to Israel [2], excessive training is rarely the only reason for overtraining. The reason is more likely due to faulty training, where the contribution of other factors to the total load has not been sufficiently considered. The most common factors for overtraining in a healthy athlete include prolonged training sessions, training at excessive exercise intensities, or leaving insufficient time for recovery.

Other important factors contributing to overtraining include other demands such as continuously working too hard, problems in human relations, incorrect eating habits, sleeplessness, various inflammations, excessive smoking and alcohol/drug intake. The significance of such factors increases when training is very intensive. Overtraining is the burn-out syndrome of athletes.

Manifestations of Overtraining

Overtraining is a state of fatigue in the entire organism but it can manifest itself in individual organs such as the heart or the musculoskeletal systems. There may also be mental disturbances such as sudden loss of trust in one's own ability, irritability, or nervousness [4].

A Psychophysiological Disturbance?

The first symptoms of overtraining vary depending on the type of sport, on the amount and type of training, on external factors, and, expecially, on individual characteristics (age, gender, state of health, physical capacity). Acccording to Dempo [3], overtraining is a state of resembling neurosis, due to excessive loading of the central nervous system and other parts of the organism. Others [5] have stated that overtraining would be primarily a manifestation of increased activity of the sympathoadrenal system.

An exceptionally significant manifestation of overtraining is disturbance in the hormonal regulation of energy and protein metabolism resulting in catabolic metabolism, i.e. reduction of muscle mass. It causes weight loss, among other things.

Sympathetic and Parasympathetic Overtraining

According to Israel [2], overtraining can be either sympathetic or parasympathetic because the effects of either autonomic nervous system may be prominent. Sympathetic nerve stimulation results in functional activation, a fight or flight reaction. Parasympathetic activation results in slowing down and recovery.

Table 1. Symptons of overtraining [2]

Sympathetic overtraining	Parasympathetic overtraining
Fatigue	Fatigue
Irritability	Calmness
Sleeplessness	Normal sleep
Lack of appetite	Normal appetite
Weight loss	No change in weight
Easy sweating	Normal regulation of body temperature
Nocturnal sweating, moist hands	
Frequent headaches	No headaches
Palpitation, heaviness and stabbing pain in the chest	–
Rapid resting pulse rate	Normal resting pulse rate
Increased basal metabolism	Normal basal metabolism
Slightly increased body temperature	Normal body temperature
Delayed recovery of pulse rate after exercise	Normal recovery of pulse rate after exercise
Faster than normal increase in breathing rate during exercise	No breathing problems
Decreased tolerance to stress	–
Poor coordination of movements	Clumsy movements and poor coordination especially during hard exercise
Shortened reaction time	Normal or lengthened reaction time
Shaky hands	–
Restlessness and/or depressed mood	Normal mood

In sympathetic, or classical, overtraining, the subject does not feel healthy. Sympathetic overtraining with its abundant symptoms is easiest to diagnose. It resembles, to some extent, hyperthyroidism, and easily results from attempts to develop one's best condition too quickly. Parasympathetic overtraining is much more difficult to diagnose because its main manifestation is disturbances in the hormonal regulation of energy and protein metabolism. Manifestations of the two types of overtraining are listed in table 1. Sympathetic overtraining is typically observed in young athletes initiating their careers, parasympathetic overtraining in more experienced athletes. Parasympathetic overtraining usually develops more slowly, and its onset is often difficult to detect. Its main symptom, decreased maximal performance, may be its only symptom. Usually the athlete will have no unusual symptoms while at rest or during moderate exercise.

The Syndrome of Heart Overstrain – Local Overtraining

A form of overtraining differing from those discussed above has been observed [6] in young athletes – the syndrome of heart overstrain (overstrain of an individual organ). In a severe case, the patient suffers from a feeling of heaviness and pain in the chest, palpitations, negative waves in ECG recordings [7] and headache. Symptoms usually disappear after interruption of training for 2–3 months.

Diagnosis of Overtraining

Overtraining is not easy to detect in its early phase. According to Heipertz [8], overtrained athletes frequently report more infections than usual (perhaps due to stress-induced immunosuppression). Infectious diseases may also be a precipating factor, because overtraining often appears after such diseases or if training is not interrupted pending a latent infection. A medical check-up should be performed to reveal current and previous infections if overtraining is suspected.

Overtraining can best be avoided by using well-programmed, systematic training methods (gradual increases in intensity/duration) and sensibly chosen physiological/biochemical tests to follow the level of physical loading at appropriate intervals during training. To prevent overtraining, it is important to make sure that there is sufficient time for recovery after training and competition.

General Symptoms

The coach is often the first to detect an athlete's performance decrement. If the athlete him-/herself suspects overtraining, it may be useful to compare amounts of training with changes in performance.

If the amount of training or loading has been notably increased and competition or laboratory loading tests still do not improve, or even get worse, further increases in the amount of training will exacerbate the problem (fig. 1).

Changes in Pulse Rate and Body Weight

The simplest and most reliable means to detect overtraining include, in addition to an analysis of training quantity and changes in performance, daily measurements of resting pulse rate and body weight.

It is a well-known fact that the resting pulse rate decreases with improving physical performance. In sympathetic overtraining, it usually increases, and recovery of resting pulse rate following exercise is delayed.

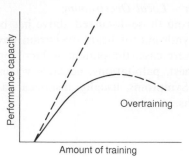

Fig. 1. Effect of amount of training on development of performance capacity and overtraining.

Furthermore, orthostatic tolerance (standing up quickly after lying down) is impaired (greater increases in pulse rate, exceeding 25 beats/min).

However, the orthostatic tolerance test has several limitations in showing overtraining. First, it is not very suitable for showing parasympathetic overtraining, and second, in young people, the result easily becomes positive and shows only existing overtraining.

Monitoring resting and recovery pulse rate as well as of changes in the orthostatic tolerance are simple tests that can be used by either athletes or their coaches to assess whether overtraining exists. If overtraining is suspected, pulse rate (60 s) should be measured during each morning (while still in bed). If it is clearly increased on several mornings relative to previous levels, the amount of training should be decreased for a while. Delayed recovery of pulse rate after training is also associated with overtraining [9]. Overtrained athletes sometimes show a decrease in maximal oxygen consumption and in duration of exercise performance time.

Body weight loss due to muscle catabolism is a late symptom of overtraining. Therefore, the simplest way to notice overtraining is regular weighing. It should be done in the stablest possible circumstances, such as every morning before breakfast, after going to the toilet. Combined with other symptoms and assuming normal hydration, weight loss on several consecutive mornings suggests overtraining.

Detection of overtraining at an initial stage or even before its actual manifestation is extremely difficult based on the currently available physiological indicators. The best approach is to closely monitor the typical features of overtraining: decreased performance, loss of desire to train, loss of appetite and increased heart rate in the morning. For a more accurate diagnosis, biochemical indicators are needed.

Changes in Testosterone and Cortisol Levels

Endogenous hormones are important for the regulation of fuel use as well as for exercise (stress) tolerance. Changes in blood hormone levels are thus also suitable for monitoring possible overtraining. This view is supported by several studies. When changes in blood testosterone levels have been studied during and after exercise, it has been observed that the heavier the loading, the greater the decrease in blood testosterone and the longer it remains depressed. With moderate exercise and sufficient recovery, no decrease can be detected in testosterone levels [10–12]. Aakvaag et al. [13] have shown that testosterone levels decrease in men during heavy physical and/or mental loading. The decrease begins on the very first day, and after a week values can approach those found in females [13]. In addition, the levels of steroid hormone binding globulin (SHBG) increase simultaneously in blood, indicating a true lack of androgenic hormones.

To be able to understand the effects of testosterone on the organism, one must also consider corticosteroids secreted by the adrenal cortex. In situations of stress, they strive to change metabolism so that the most effective source of energy, glucose, is prepared from other energy sources in the organism (proteins). Like other steroids, corticosteroids circulate in the bloodstream free or bound to a protein (corticosteroid-binding globulin, CBG). The free hormone can get into a cell and prevent protein synthesis there. Such a state where building blocks of the organism (proteins) are decomposed faster than they are produced is called catabolism. In clinical medicine, this is commonly seen, for example, in connection with surgery, severe traumas, infections and undernourishment. Overtraining caused by excessive training appears to be similar.

When blood corticosteroid levels have been monitored during physical loading, it has been observed that the heavier the strain, the more the levels increase and the longer they remain elevated after the performance [11]. In speed and power events, especially, athletes have to train very hard during certain training periods. If such training is repeated daily without sufficient recovery (light training), blood testosterone levels may stay low and cortisol levels high for long periods. This type of training will cause, in the long run, tiring and weakening of muscles and of the whole organism, i.e. chronic catabolism, because the anabolic effect of testosterone is thus minimal and the catabolic effect of cortisol maximal. Long hard training can induce an imbalance between anabolic (androgens) and catabolic hormones (corticosteroids), i.e. a clear decrease in the testosterone/cortisol ratio [14] (fig. 2). During recovery after hard training androgen secretion into the bloodstream decreases to such an extent that protein metabolism cannot turn anabolic. As a result there is no countereffect to the catabolic effects of corticosteroids on muscle cells.

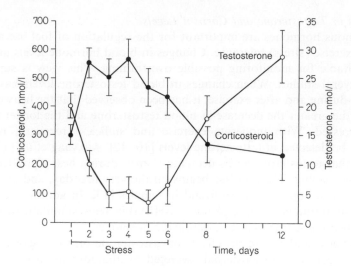

Fig. 2. Long hard training (stress) induces an imbalance between anabolic (testosterone) and catabolic (corticosteroid) hormones.

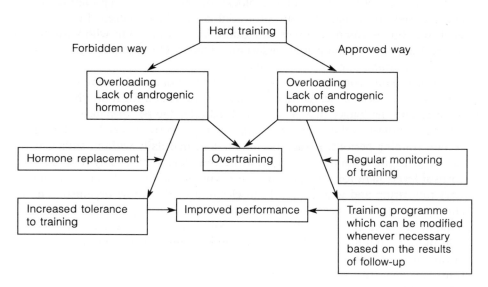

Fig. 3. Performance capacity can be increased in two ways. In the approved way, increase is based on knowledge of one's capacity and responsibility for training with regular monitoring.

Figure 3 shows two alternatives for avoiding catabolism, due to overtraining. As the left section of the figure shows, the amount of training can be increased if the decrease in blood testosterone level due to hard training is counteracted, e.g. by taking exogenous testosterone. Overtraining can thus be 'treated' with drugs making it possible to train harder than normal. However, this is considered doping and as such forbidden. Another acceptable way is depicted to the right in figure 3. Here, training and its effects are monitored by determining testosterone and cortisol levels. In this way, excessive loading can be detected before overtraining occurs.

Blood testosterone and SHBG levels can be measured and the index of biologically active free testosterone calculated on the basis of these values (table 4). Cortisol levels can also be determined in urine. However, utilization of this method is complicated by the fact that it is difficult to obtain complete urine specimens gathered over long periods of time. This method also has problems because muscle work increases creatine secretion in urine. An extremely interesting alternative method is to determine both testosterone and cortisol levels in saliva; as it has been shown that the salivary levels of both correlate well with levels of the free, i.e. active, hormones in the blood [15–17].

Indicators of Muscle Catabolism

Fats and carbohydrates are the primary sources of energy but part of the amino acids released from decomposing proteins are also used for energy production. New tissue proteins can only be formed of amino acids. Some of these amino acids are indispensable, i.e. must be obtained via diet. Therefore, in a catabolic state, i.e. where there is already overtraining, proteins hold a critical position. The amount of protein decreases when a significant quantity of amino acids are used for energy production. The result is weight loss, because the organism starts to 'consume' itself.

In clinical medicine, attempts to diagnose catabolism concentrate mainly on assessing changes in visceral (structural proteins in the viscera, and plasma proteins formed in the liver) and somatic proteins (structural proteins in the muscles and in the skeleton). Unfortunately, most methods typically used in clinical medicine are not sensitive enough to overtraining induced catabolism, i.e. measures of body weight, arm or leg circumferences, serum albumin, etc. react too slowly and are affected by many other factors.

Determination of the serum prealbumin level is considered to be the most sensitive and useful indicator of the state of visceral protein mass. The biological half-life of prealbumin in plasma is only 2–3 days [18], and therefore it reacts quickly to changes in visceral protein mass. In addition, changes in the hormonal balance do not affect the level of prealbumin as they do those of many other plasma proteins.

Urinary creatine levels have long been used as reflecting the amount of somatic protein mass [19]. Creatine is produced in connection with the metabolism of muscular phosphocreatine and does not itself undergo any metabolism before being excreted in the urine. Its excretion thus roughly reflects the amount of muscle mass. Determination of urinary creatine as such is easy, the greatest problems being posed by inaccuracy in urine sampling and by the fact that the heavy muscle work can increase the excretion of creatine in urine. Finally, creatine is a relatively insensitive variable.

Urinary N-methylhistidine (3-methylhistidine) excretion theoretically is an excellent marker of somatic protein breakdown. It forms in muscle tissues as a modification product after the syntheses of actin and myosin. The human body cannot utilize the 3-methylhistidine released as the two proteins are decomposed, and it is therefore excreted in urine, 95% in an unchanged and 5% in an acetylated form [20]. There is relatively little 3-methylhistidine in other proteins in the body, more than 95% being in muscular actomyosin [21]. One of the main obstacles for routine use of 3-methylhistidine is the difficulty of its measurement. This usually involves high-pressure liquid or ion-exchange chromatography which might be useful in the study of overtraining in athletes.

Excretion of zinc in the urine has been observed to increase easily in catabolism [22]. At present, the theoretical background of this phenomenon is inadequately understood. However, in catabolic states zinc excretion has been shown to follow closely that of 3-methylhistidine [23], and it therefore seems reasonable that this zinc would be derived from muscle tissue.

Appearance in blood of an enzyme specific for skeletal muscles, creatine kinase (CK-MM), suggests that muscle cells are damaged to some extent. The more severe the damage the more enzyme there should be in blood. Determination of blood CK-MM level may be significant for the determination of muscle catabolism. Measurement of the total activity is sufficient for routine analysis, because most CK activity in blood is derived from muscle tissue. After a marathon run, for instance, CK levels are several times higher than basal values [24]. The better condition of the athlete, the smaller the increase in CK level. However, although enzyme efflux undoubtedly indicates some damage, the actual relationship between damage as assessed via election micrographs and enzyme efflux is not very good [25].

Experimental Approach to Monitor Overtraining

With this in mind, we exposed a group of young long-distance runners to intense training for 1 week whereafter they were examined using various

Table 2. The appearance of overtraining in the normal training group

Subject No.	Orthostatic test			Resting pulse rate beats/min	Recovery after maximal exercise pulse rate, beats/min		Diagnosis
	pulse rate	blood pressure	ECG changes		maximum	10 min after	
13	−	−	−	54	180	98	non-overtraining
4	−	−	−	67	175	98	non-overtraining
10	−	−	−	52	175	98	non-overtraining
2	−	−	−	40	176	86	non-overtraining
8	−	−	−	64	unable to run on treadmill		uncertain
6	−	−	+	68	170	105	overtraining

Overtraining: an abnormal orthostatic test with a positive pulse (increase >25 min^{-1}), blood pressure (systolic increase >5 mm Hg, diastolic increase >20 mm Hg) or ECG reaction (T-wave inversion in leads 2, aVF, 3, V_5, V_6) and slowed recovery (pulse rate >100 beats/min ten min after the exercise).
Non-overtraining: A normal orthostatic test and normal recovery.

Table 3. The appearance of overtraining in the hard training group

Subject No.	Orthostatic test			Resting pulse rate beats/min	Recovery after maximal exercise pulse rate, beats/min		Diagnosis
	pulse rate	blood pressure	ECG changes		maximum	10 min after	
11	+	−	−	52	175	102	overtraining
16	+	−	−	53	170	102	overtraining
14	+	−	−	53	200	130	overtraining
7	+	−	−	50	185	100	overtraining
3	+	−	−	70	162	108	overtraining
5	−	−	+	67	176	95	uncertain
1	+	−	−	42	170	81	uncertain
12	+	−	−	47	175	85	uncertain
15	−	−	−	48	192	83	non-overtraining

Overtraining: An abnormal orthostatic test with a positive pulse, blood pressure or ECG reaction and slowed recovery (pulse rate >100 beats/min 10 min after the exercise).
Uncertain: Either normal reactions in the orthostatic test with slow recovery or vice versa.
Non-overtraining: A normal orthostatic test and normal recovery.

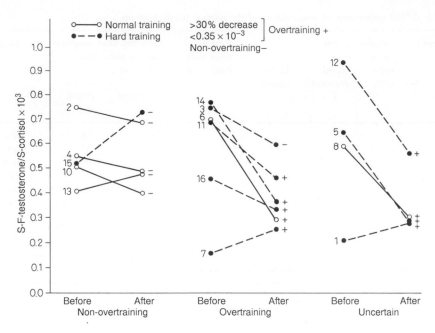

Fig. 4. Comparison of physiological and biochemical testing in the normal and hard training group.

physiological and biochemical tests to detect possible overtraining [9]. Runners of similar age and training status served as the control group.

The results of physiological testing in the control group (regular training) are shown in table 2. On the right side of the table, the diagnosis is given according to the criteria shown in the footnote. Overtraining in the hard training group is depicted in table 3. Five of the subjects were in overtraining, 3 were grouped as uncertain and one clearly as non-overtraining.

According to this physiological testing the subjects were grouped into three caterories: non-overtraining, overtraining and uncertain, as seen in figure 4. Biochemically, overtraining was diagnosed when the serum-free testosterone/serum cortisol ratio was less than 0.35×10^{-3} or if the decrease after the training period was more than 30% of the starting value (marked 'plus' in figure 4). For all subjects in the non-overtraining group the biochemical testing agreed with the physiological testing (these subjects were marked 'minus', fig. 4). The physiological overtraining group contained one subject (No. 3) who, according to biochemical testing, was regarded as non-overtraining and therefore marked 'minus'. All subjects in the physiologically uncertain group were biochemically regarded as

Table 1 Patterns of overtraining using different biochemical indices

Physiological assessment	Non-overtraining					Overtraining						Uncertain			
Biochemical indices	No. 2	No. 4	No. 10	No. 13	No. 15	No. 3	No. 6	No. 7	No. 11	No. 14	No. 16	No. 1	No. 5	No. 8	No. 12
S-F-testosterone/S-cortisol[1]	–	–	–	–	–	–	+	+	+	+	+	+	+	+	+
S-testosterone/S-cortisol[2]	–	–	+	–	–	–	+	+	+	+	+	+	+	+	–
S-SHBG[3]	+	–	–	–	–	–	+	+	–	+	+	+	–	+	+
S-HGH[4]	–	–	–	–	+	–	+	+	–	+	+	–	–	–	–
S-prealbumin[5]	–	–	–	–	+	–	–	–	–	+	+	–	–	–	–
S-CK	–	+	–	–	–	–	+	–	+	–	–	–	+	+	–
U-3-methylhistidine[7]	–	–	–	–	–	–	+	n.d.	–	–	–	–	+	+	–
Sa-testosterone/Sa-cortisol[8]	+	–	+	–	+	–	+	n.d.	–	+	–	–	+	+	–

S = Serum; U = urine; Sa = Saliva; F = Free; n.d. = not determined.
Criteria for diagnosing overtraining biochemically (the subject in overtraining indicated by "plus").
[1] $< 0.5 \times 10^{-3}$ or more than 30% decrease.
[2] $< 0.30 \times 10^{-1}$ or more than 30% decrease.
[3] > 3 nmol/l or more than 50% increase.
[4] > 0 µg/l.
[5] < 0 mg/l or more than 30% decrease.
[6] > 3 U/l or more than 50% increase.
[7] > 50 µmol/l or more than 50% increase.
[8] $< 10 \times 10^{-1}$ or more than 30% decrease.

overtrained and, therefore, marked 'plus'. This may be because hormonal changes in the blood occur in the early phase of overtraining.

Table 4 provides a summary of our results in diagnosing overtraining with the various clinical chemical tests. The criteria for the biochemical diagnosis of overtraining in various tests are given in the footnote to the table. When the serum total testosterone/serum cortisol ratio was used as the biochemical marker of overtraining, 1 subject (No. 10) in the physiological non-overtrained group was regarded as overtraining and therefore marked 'plus'. One subject (No. 3) in the physiological overtraining group was regarded as non-overtraining and therefore marked 'minus'.

When the serum growth hormone test was applied to the diagnosis of overtraining, 3 of 6 subjects in the physiological overtraining group showed high values, between 10 and 20 μg/l, after the training period.

Serum prealbumin, serum creatine kinase, urine 3-methylhistidine and saliva testosterone/saliva cortisol ratio gave inconsistent results in classifying overtraining.

Treatment of Overtraining

Overtrained athletes and those heading towards overtraining should be 'treated' according to the following guidelines:

(1) Factors leading to obvious overtraining should be determined and elimated. Here, attention should be paid to other factors in daily life as well as to factors related to training.

(2) During overtraining, recovery should be sufficiently emphasized as opposed to loading. Thus, the intensity and the amount of training should be clearly reduced for a while.

(3) Adequate quantity and quality of nutrition should be ensured regardless of any loss of appetite connected with overtraining. Regular sleep is also very important.

(4) Training with monotonous loading should be avoided. A change in the training environment or even a change of event for a while may be required.

Conclusion

According to various studies and observations overtraining is considered a state where, despite continuous training, performance often fails to improve or even decrease. It is due to physical and mental overloading and may develop regardless of ostensibly correct training. Overloading of the organism produces disturbances in nervous and hormonal regulation.

Sympathetic overtraining in young or novice athletes is relatively easy to detect due to abundant symptomatology including increased resting pulse rate, prolonged recovery of pulse rate following exercise, sympathetic orthostatic intolerance, and weight loss. The diagnosis of parasympathetic overtraining in elite and experienced athletes, on the other hand, is rarely diagnosed without metabolic and hormonal measures. These are seen as clear decrease in serum free testosterone/cortisol ratio. Prevention should involve regular monitoring of symptoms including laboratory rests, gradual increases in the amount of training according to development of performance capacity, adequate recovery, and elimination of environmental factors disturbing training.

References

1   Karvonen J, Härkönen M: Urheilijan ylikunto. Suom Lääkäril 1983;38:2330–2334.
2   Israel S: Zur Problematik des Uebertrainings aus internistischer und leistungsphysiologischer Sicht. Med Sport 1976;16:1–10.
3   Dempo A: Some clinical problems in modern sports medicine. XXIIth World Congr Sports Medicine, Vienna, July 1982, Abstracts volume.
4   Karvonen J: Ylirasitus ja sen toteaminen. VK-lehti 1986;11:26–27.
5   Silujanova VA, Sokova EV, Bolshakova TD, Alaverdjan AM, Alperovich BR, Gorodetsky VV: Complex study of earlier stages of chronic physical overstrain. XXIIth World Congr Sports Medicine, Vienna, July 1982, Abstracts volume.
6   Badridze NM, Bogdanov JN: Rehabilitation of young athletes with the syndrome of heart overstrain. XXIIth World Congr Sports Medicine, Vienna, July, 1982, Abstracts volume.
7   Hanne-Paparo N, Drory Y, Schoenfeld Y, Shapira J, Kellerman JJ: Common ECG changes in athletes. Cardiology 1976;61:267–278.
8   Heipertz W: Training und Trainingsformen; in: Sportsmedizin. Stuttgart, Thieme, 1980, pp 57–58.
9   Härkönen M, Kuoppasalmi K, Näveri H, Tikkanen H, Icén A, Adlercreutz H, Karvonen J: Biochemical indicators in diagnosis of overstrain condition in athletes. Biomechanics-Kinanthropometry and Sports Medicine, Exercise Science. Olympic Scientific Congress, Eugene, July 1984.
10 Dessypris A, Kuoppasalmi K, Adlercreutz H: Plasma cortisol, testosterone, androstendione and luteinizing hormone (LH) in a non-competitive marathon run. J Steroid Biochem. 1976;7:33–37.
11 Kuoppasalmi K, Näveri H, Härkönen, M. Adlercreutz H: Plasma cortisol, androstendione, testorone and luteinizing hormone in running exercise of different intensities. Scand J Clin Lab Invest 1980;40:403–409.
12 Kuoppasalmi K: Effects of exercise stress on human plasma hormone levels with special reference to steroid hormones; academic Diss, University of Helsinki, 1981, pp 1–54.
13 Aakvaag A, Dentdal Ø, Quigatad K, Wolstad P, Rønningen H, Fonnum F: Testosterone and testosterone binding globulin (TeBG) in young men during prolonged stress. Int J Androl 1978;1:22–31.

14   Adlercreutz H, Härkönen M, Kuoppasalmi K, Näveri H, Huhtaniemi I, Tikkanen H, Remes K, Dessypris A, Karvonen J: Effect of training on plasma anabolic and catabolic steroid hormones and their response during physical exercise. Int J Sports Med 1986;7:27–28.

15   Walker RF, Riad-Fahmy D, Read GF: Adrenal status assessed by direct radioimmunoassay of cortisol in whole saliva or parotid saliva. Clin Chem 1978;24:1460–1463.

16   Walker RF, Wilson DW, Read GF, Riad-Fahmy D: Assessment of testicular function by the radioimmunoassay of testosterone in saliva. Int J Androl 1980;3:105–120.

17   Umeda T, Hiramtsu R, Iwaoka T, Shimada T, Miura F, Sato T: Use of saliva for monitoring unbound free cortisol levels in serum. Clin Chim Acta 1981;110:245–253.

18   Ingenbleek Y, van den Schrieck HG, de Nayer P, de Visscher M: Albumin, transferrin and the thyroxine-binding prealbumin/retinol-binding protein (TBPA-RBP) complex in assessment of malnutrition. Clin Chim Acta 1975;63:61–67.

19   Forbes GB, Bruining GJ: Urinary creatinine excretion and lean body mass. Am J Clin Nutr 1976;29:1359–1366.

20   Long CL, Haverberg LN, Young VT, Kinney JM, Munro HN, Geiger JW: Metabolism of 3-methylhistidine in man. Metabolism 1975;24:929–935.

21   Munro HN, Young VR: Urinary excretion of 3-methylhistidine: A tool to study metabolic responses in relation to nutrition and hormonal status in health and disease of man. Am J Clin Nutr 1978;31:1608–1614.

22   Warhold I: Metodik vid bestämning av nutritionsstatus. Näringsforskning 1981;25:1–140.

23   Warhold I, Isaksson B, Sandström B, Hultén L, Magnusson O: Nutritional status after major bowel surgery – the effect of nutritional support. Vår Föda 1979;31(suppl 3).

24   Remes K: Veritutkimuksetko avuksi palautumisen selvittelyssä. Valmennus 1982;7:16–17.

25   Evans, WJ, Cannon JG: The metabolic effects of exercise-induced muscle damage. Exerc Sport Sci Rev 1991;19:103–104.

Dr. Juha Karvonen, National Agency for Welfare and Health,
P.O. Box 220, SF-00531 Helsinki (Finland)

Karvonen J, Lemon PWR, Iliev I (eds): Medicine in Sports Training and Coaching.
Med Sport Sci. Basel, Karger, 1992, vol 35, pp 189–214

Importance of Warm-Up and Cool Down on Exercise Performance

Juha Karvonen

Department of Clinical Physiology, University Hospital of Tampere, Finland

Contents

Introduction

Prior to particularly heavy physical exercises most individuals engage in some type of warm-up activity; however, frequently this occurs without any systematic plan. In contrast with elite athletes, warm-up is a critical part of their preparation because it has been shown to positively influence performance. Unfortunately, the actual warm-up methods used are usually based on the trial and error experience of the athlete or the coach rather than on scientific study.

The major aims of warm-up are to achieve better results in the subsequent athletic performance and to minimize the chances of incurring an injury. Methods of warm-up can be either active, with one performing muscular exercise during which metabolism increases, or passive, using massage or primarily passive mechano- or thermotherapeutic procedures.

Active warm-up usually consists of various physical exercises, such as stretching, jumping, and/or running. Through these exercises an effort is made to improve the performance capacity of the locomotion and metabolic systems (general warm-up). Before participating in athletic performances demanding general concentration, steadiness, coordination, fine muscle movements, and/or complex skills it is also useful to repeat important movements (specific warming-up).

In order to maximize the benefits of warm-up, one should design warm-up procedures as closely as possible to the kind of activity to be performed, as well as to the individual athlete. This requires a thorough understanding of both the athletic event and the athlete. When the specific programme is created it must be based on known physiological principles. Factors such as the exercise intensity and duration and whether the warm-up consists of intermittent or continuous exercise may be critical.

Physiological Basis

Body Temperature

Clearly observable adaptation phenomena are known to occur during warm-up. One of these is the increase in body temperature. From a physiological point of view it is not clear, whether warm-up causes any favourable effects on physical performance, though certain physiological changes in the circulatory and oxygen transport systems and in mobilization of various hormones are caused by an increase in body temperature [1].

About 100 years ago observations of how muscular exercise increases body temperature were published. Subsequent studies using different kinds of materials and subjects have been reported [4–6].

Today it is known that a muscle functions as a 'chemodynamic engine' that transforms chemical energy into mechanical work and at the same time produces large quantities of heat. The increase of body temperature with exercise is due to heat production by the active muscles and, therefore, depends upon both exercise intensity and duration.

This body temperature increase improves one's performance capacity in many ways. At the beginning of this century Zuntz et al. [7, 8] mentioned the disappearance of the subjective feeling of stiffness following warm-up. When the body temperature is increasing, transmission of nerve impulses, nerve and muscle irritability, contractility and power output of a muscle also increase [9]. Many investigators [10–14] have found that the mechanical efficiency (work completed/energy utilized) of a muscle improves when body temperature increases. In addition, Asmussen and Böje [12] found that subjects (numbers 2–4) could complete a certain amount of work in a shorter time subsequent to an increase in muscular temperature.

Observations made by Kleitman et al. [15] demonstrate that reaction time for visual and auditory stimuli varies directly with the diurnal body temperature curve. These studies found the poorest reaction early in the morning and late at night, when body temperature was lowest. Though there seemed to be a distinct relationship between the changes in body temperature and reaction time, these investigators did not consider the decrease in reaction time and the improvement of physical performance capacity to be due only to increased body temperature. That is, reaction time might be affected also by factors other than body temperature.

An increase of body temperature by 1 °C increases metabolic rate by about 13% [16]. During exercise, body temperature increases are determined primarily by the exercise intensity relative to the individual's capacity and remain proportionally constant independent of the changes in the air temperature, humidity and air flow [11, 17].

Passive warm-up also increases body temperature. The effect of passive warm-up on competition results has been tested by some investigators, who have used hot showers, warm baths, massage or diathermy [14, 18, 19]. In general these procedures do not have beneficial effects on the exercise results.

Evaporation of sweat in response to passive heating [20] as well as to exercise [21] plays an important role in increase of body temperature. Chwalbinska-Moneta and Hänninen [22] have demonstrated that warm-up results in a sudden rise in sweat rate which subsequently minimizes the exercise hyperthermia. Regular endurance training results in an earlier onset of sweating (>sweat rate at a given body temperature) which further reduces the chances of hyperthermia.

Energy Metabolism

The increase in metabolism causes greater need for oxygen. Under aerobic conditions the necessary oxygen is provided to the active muscles by increase in respiration and circulation. When the exercise is very intense oxygen delivery is inadequate, despite these changes, and anaerobic energy utilization increases. According to several studies, the metabolism of a trained subject adjusts more easily to an increased need for energy than an untrained subject. Those studies have found that at the same absolute workload muscle blood flow and heart rate of those trained remains lower than of those untrained.

Carbohydrates (liver and muscle glycogen) release through anaerobic glycolysis the greatest part of the energy needed in a heavy physical exercise of short durations (e.g. runs of 200–800 m). The end-product of this process is lactic acid. When the physical exercise is longer and the workload lower the contribution of anaerobic glycolysis is replaced by aerobic energy production (utilizing both carbohydrate and fat and perhaps some protein for energy). Contributing to this are increased glucagon and epinephrine which, by activating adenyl cyclase, increase mobilisation of carbohydrate from the liver into blood. Insulin assists the entry of glucose into the functioning muscular cell; however, this may be unnecessary because exercise improves glucose transport and utilization.

During warm-up the glucose needed for starting muscular function is liberated from liver glycogen by sympathetic stimulation. Physical exercise increases the concentration of norepinephrine in plasma more than the concentration of epinephrine, which suggests that the sympathetic nervous system is stimulated to a greater extent than the adrenal glands. In addition, anticipation of the subsequent competition would be expected to cause a sympathetic outflow, even without warming up. Moreover, prior strenuous short-term exercise in addition to the increase in blood glucose, plasma insulin can increase threefold from 24.6 to 75.6 mU/l. This should increase the use of blood glucose as an energy source, because of the favourable effect of insulin on glucose uptake by the muscle cell.

If disturbances in glycolysis occur, physical performance capacity suffers. One of the factors limiting performance capacity is the final product from anaerobic glycolysis, lactic acid. The increase of muscle lactic acid concentration during exercise slows glycolysis by inhibiting the activity of glycolytic enzymes, such as phosphofructokinase [23] and lactate dehydrogenase [24].

Margaria et al. [25, 26] have endeavoured to show that blood lactic acid concentration does not significantly increase during running, if the running is so light that aerobic energy regeneration equals the rate of energy utilization. Cobb and Johnson [27] emphasized that during exercise lactic and pyruvic acid increase less in those trained than in those untrained, though those untrained have not been able to perform nearly the same amount of physical exercise during the test. Even at workloads < 50% VO_2 max (50% of the maximum oxygen up-take) an increase blood lactic acid concentration can occur in nonathletes [28]. In athletes the corresponding increase appeared at workloads > 60–65% $\dot{V}O_2$ max. While running on the threadmill at 67–74% $\dot{V}O_2$ max the lactic acid concentration of venous blood increased from 8.0 to 29 mg% (0.9 and 3.4 mmol/l) in nonathletes. Keul [29] suggested that the workload that increases blood lactic acid concentration to 4 mmol/l (OBLA = onset of blood lactate accumulation) be considered the threshold between aerobic and anaerobic performance. The blood lactic acid concentration should not exceed this level at the end of warm-up. In a study on endurance runners and skiers performed by Karvonen [30], warm-up caused only a slight increase in the lactic acid concentration of venous blood, which did not return to its basal level before the start of competition.

Using limited material Asmussen and Böje [12] have published results showing that subsequent to warm-up less oxygen is needed to perform a certain amount of physical work. In addition, Yamaguchi [31] found that following warm-up $\dot{V}O_2$ max is slightly higher than during strenuous physical exercise performed without warm-up. Saltin [32] reported that during athletic performances lasting only a few minutes $\dot{V}O_2$ max remains 5% lower if warm-up was inadequate.

At the onset exercise oxygen uptake ($\dot{V}O_2$) increases toward steady state more rapidly in trained than in untrained persons [33]. Following the onset of mild to moderate intensity exercise, the time course of rise of $\dot{V}O_2$ is principally dictated by the intramuscular process underlying aerobic energy production and by changes in body O_2 stores. It is likely that warm-up increases the kinetics of the cardiorespiratory response to exercise and decreases the exercise-induced body lactate accumulation [34].

Respiration

It is known that respiration is controlled by neural (fast) and humoral (slow) components. The fast component controls the changes in respiratory function at the very beginning of the performance. With respect to warm-up very little scientific attention has been directed toward ventilation, perhaps because the exercise intensity is relatively low. During physical exercise of similar intensity to warm-up, Wigertz [35] found that respiration rate increases very quickly. According to Paulev [36], the second and third breaths can be performed as early as 5–10 s from the start of the performance. The investigations carried out by Ekelund [37, 38] show that the respiration rate and minute volume of all the test subjects levelled off during the first 10 min. When Yamaguchi [13] compared pulmonary ventilation between step test performances with and without warm-up, he found that ventilation was lower following warm-up. According to Karvonen [30], the respiratory response to high intensity exercise was the same regardless of warm-up.

In their classical work Barcroft and King [39] mentioned that oxygen is more completely dissociated from hemoglobin due to the increase of temperature in the tissues caused by physical exercise. A similar effect results from the exercise-included increases in pCO_2, lactic acid, and 2,3-DPG [40, 42]. This means that as a result of warm-up the blood releases oxygen to tissues more easily [41]. Brundin [43] observed a significant correlation ($r = 0.92$) between the rise in pulmonary artery blood temperature during exercise and the increase in the arteriovenous (a-v) oxygen difference. In this study a linear relationship between the increase of pulmonary artery blood temperature and a-v oxygen difference was found until 1 °C so that increase of 0.5 °C increases a-v oxygen difference 50 ml/l and 1 °C increase 100 ml/l.

Circulation

Ramsey et al. [44] reported that heart rates vary markedly during different phases of warm-up prior to playing basketball. On the other hand, when the exercise intensity is controlled heart rate also remains comparatively constant [37, 38, 45, 46]. Heart rate increases very quickly at the beginning of strenuous calisthenics or with exercises frequently used in warm-up and after that it varies depending on the subsequent exercise intensity.

Using the serial of 10 jumps with boys (aged 12–14 years), Klint and Nitschke [47] observed increased heart rates from 103–112 to 168–171 bpm. With 12- to 14-year old girls, who had rested 20 min immediately prior to a 60-meter dash, resting heat rates just prior to the start of the race changed from 125 to 141 bpm. The sudden increase of heart rate in young persons like this is obviously more a consequence of vegetative tonus changes.

At the starting point of the contests the increase in heart rate is elevated by increased sympathetic stimulation caused by excitement. In experiments performed with endurance athletes Karvonen [30] has observed that warm-up causes increased heart rate, which did not return to resting values before the start of competition. Further, with heavy physical

Table 1. Physiological effects of warm-up

Circulation and the oxygen transport system are more ready for heavy exercise

Release of oxygen from hemoglobin and myoglobin is increased

Muscular blood flow is increased

Muscular performance capacity is increased and muscular viscosity is decreased

Transmission of nerve impulses is increased and the sensitivity of nerve receptors is increased

Neuromuscular coordination improves

Predisposition to muscular, tendon and connective tissue injuries decreases

---

exercise, heart rate reached steady state more quickly following warm-up than without it. However, Chwalbinska-Moneta and Hänninen [22] failed to find any change in the circulatory, ventilatory, or metabolic response to exercise regardless of whether or not warm-up occurred. In addition, in untrained males Knowlton et al. [48] were unable to find any significant differences between heart rate, lactic acid, and oxygen uptake due to warm-up. Finally, results obtained by De Bruyn-Provost [49] did not conclusively show a positive effect of warm-up before exercise.

The marked effect of excitement and changes in mood on heart rate has also been observed in nonsport settings. Using telemetry Clasing et al. [50] and Christian and Spohr [51] measured higher heart rates of aviation students during flight and of patients in the psychiatrist's office at different phases of conversation with their doctor.

Long-term training is known to decrease resting heart rate, but according to the experiments carried out by Brundin and Cernigliaro [52] it does not change the cooperation between the sympathetic nerve system and the adrenal glands. The urinary output of catecholamines correlates with physical strain in that the excretion of norepinephrine increases markedly when exercise intensity exceeds 70% $\dot{V}O_2$ max. On the other hand, Pavlik [53] has reported that the same physical strain causes smaller excretion of catecholamines in athletes as in nonathletes (table 1).

The dead point-second wind phenomena seem to be related to adjustments in the circulation system at the beginning of physical exercise. When athletes start continuous exercise performances of 1–30 min without appropriate warm-up they may initially feel unusual fatigue, or sharp chest pain and dyspnoea that ceases with continued performance. The former feeling is called 'dead point' and the latter 'second wind'.

Meythaler [54] suggests that the dead point is due to the decrease in blood glucose frequently observed at the beginning of intense exercise and the subsequent increase in blood glucose concentration corresponds to second wind. The increase of the blood lactic acid concentration and the decrease of pH also seem to have an effect on the occurrence of dead point.

Clear correlations between the adaptions of the respiratory and circulatory system to physical exercise and the occurrence of dead point have been observed by Ruosteenoja [5]. In these investigations carried out an healthy male medical students hyperventilation and significant increase in heart rate and rectal temperature were associated with dead point. During second wind the changes in question were nonsignificant. Blood pressure had time to become stabilised corresponding to the exercise intensity prior to dead point.

It has been stated [30] that systolic blood pressure and muscular blood flow in the lower limbs return to resting level within 4–6 min after warm-up, but during this time rectal temperature remains higher than at rest before warm-up. With intense exercise the concentration of blood glucose and lactic acid increase to the same level regardless of warm-up. Karvonen [30] concluded that for endurance athletes warm-up is beneficial for performance.

Psychological Basis

Psychological effects of warm-up have received considerably less attention than physiological ones. A reason for this might be that psychological experiments are more difficult to organize and standardize. However, some attempts have been made. Malarecki [55] has observed improved results in some sports performances using imagined warm-up. The effect of conventional warm-up on increasing performance capacity and psychological readiness has been emphasized by Puni [56].

In preparing for competitions athletes spend their time not only in achieving physical readiness but also in concentration, attempting to either discharge or increase their aggression [57]. According to Schmidt [58] elite athletes frequently experience a certain amount of frustration just prior to a contest. This frustration may be felt in different ways by each athlete. In Schmidt's opinion the best way to discharge frustration is with physical activity in which the aim is to avoid excessive passiveness, hypochondria tendencies and overemphasized activity. The physical activities connected with warm-up thus offer a suitable outlet channel. The positive or negative attitudes of the subjects prior to the test presumably have a marked effect on investigation results concerning warm-up. This could explain the results of Smith and Bozymowski [59] in which they observed that the subjects

Table 2. Psychological effects of warm-up

Positive attitude to warm-up increases positive effects

Positive effects can be removed with hypnosis

During warm-up technical and tactical details can be planned in advance

Mental training and concentration may help

---

who had a favourable attitude towards warm-up were able to improve their performance capacity markedly with warm-up. Whereas for those taking a less favourable stand, warm-up did not improve their performance.

Everybody who has participated in sports has observed warm-up to have clear psychological effects. These psychological aspects are, however, very difficult to study and as a result the literature is somewhat inadequate in the psychological area. In order to eliminate the effect of psychological factors Massey et al. [60] had their subjects perform warm-up and the subsequent exercise in a state of deep hypnosis. The same test was repeated in a deep hypnotic state without warming up. The purpose of this was to create a condition where those participating did not know whether they had warmed up or not. No differences were observed between the results of these two conditions (table 2).

A subject's level of arousal is known to influence performance. According to Yerker-Dodson [61], complex performances are enhanced if arousal can be alleviated, while simple performances are improved when arousal is increased. Perhaps warm-up could be used either to alleviate or to enhance arousal depending on the type of performance to follow.

Endurance running is a relatively simple activity. Therefore, performance should be enhanced if arousal is high before competition. Conversely, pole vaulting is quite complex, and a high level of pre-event arousal should impair the performance. The pole vaulter should also be able to relax while concentrating on his performance. In complex performances young athletes are more negatively affected by a high level of arousal than are older or more experienced athletes. The young individual has to concentrate more on the basic mechanics than does the older one. This may mean that experienced athletes will benefit from high pre-event arousal even in complex performances because at their skill level the event has become a simple activity.

According to Oxendine [62], arousal has the following effects on the different types of sport:

(1) A high level of arousal is useful in sports requiring strength, speed, and endurance.

(2) A high level of arousal impairs the performance in sports requiring skill, coordination and concentration, or a complex series of movements.

(3) A moderate level of arousal is useful in all sports.

It is not easy to know when the optimal level of arousal has been reached. Corcoran [63] suggests that the appropriate level can be determined by increasing or decreasing arousal and observing the changes in performance. If performance deteriorates when arousal is increased, the original performance was already optimal.

In team sports, and occasionally also in individual sports, certain movements and patterns of movement are performed during warm-up to frighten the opponent. These 'shows' may be successful in some situations, but anyone with an ability to concentrate and a high level of self-confidence is immune to them. The most important thing is to get oneself ready for the contest by concentrating on one's own performance instead of attempting to bluff the opponent.

A show of this kind may, however, help to warm-up the audience and to create a sympathy for the team.

Methods of Warm-Up

The warm-up procedure depends on the specificity of the movements required by different sports, i.e. whether they require static (isometric) or dynamic (isotonic) muscular work. In alpine skiing, for example, one can expect a large contribution of static effort, whereas for running the effort is mainly dynamic. It is not clear, however, whether endurance training, i.e. dynamic warm-up, can bring any positive effect for static performances and vice versa.

Active Warm-Up

According to Högberg and Ljunggren [64], the usefulness of warm-up depends upon the intensity and duration of the exercise used as well as the amount of time between the end of warm-up and start of the competition. To warm-up prior to the types of sports where speed, skill and explosive strength are needed, it might be best to concentrate on performing the actual movements as flawlessly as possible.

The effect of warm-up on 60–1760 yard runs was investigated by Simonson et al. [10], Blank [65], Mathews and Snyder [66] and Grodjinowski and Magel [67]. Active warm-up was found to improve the times

Table 3. Methods and effects of warm-up

Active warm-up	Passive warm-up
The aim of active warm-up is to improve the physical and psychic performance level by means of active muscular activity	In passive warm-up external means are used to increase body temperature
General warm-up	*Methods*
To increase body temperature	Sauna, showers, liniments
To increase blood flow to the muscle	massage
To reduce muscle viscosity	
To increase transmission of nerve impulses	
Specific warming up	*Effects*
Repetition of movements important for the sport event and competition	Blood flow is directed away from muscles
Improvement of neuromuscular coordination	Generally no positive effects on performance capacity
Mental training	An exception might be massage, which saves energy
Transitional warm-up	

significantly in some cases. For example, Mathews and Snyder [66] did not observe significant improvement for 400-yard runs following warm-up. In contrast, Grodjinowski and Magel [67] observed improvements following warm-up in 60-, 440-, and 1,760-yard (1 mile) runs. In the 60-yard run, the improvement was 2.5%. Vigorous warm-up was markedly more effective than regular warm-up (calisthenics). Vigorous warm-up improved the mile time on the average by 8.1 s.

Due to small differences in results it is likely difficult to show statistical improvement with warm-up in short sprints. Pyke [68] reported that 60-yard run times did not improve significantly subsequent to warm-up. Karpovich and Hale [18] tested the effect of warm-up (bicycle ergometer) on 440-yard run times and observed no treatment effect.

Högberg and Ljunggren [64] have suggested that endurance runners should warm-up for 15 min at 12–14 km/h running speed or 3.0–3.4 litres/min oxygen uptake ($\dot{V}O_2$). In sprints they stated that a 5-min warm-up was less effective than a 15-min warm-up, but warming up for longer than 15 min did not improve 100-meter run times. Masterovoi [69] used 4 or 5 m/s (14.4 or 18 km/h) mean running speed during warm-up and found improvement in short distance running results.

Ingjer and Strömme [34] presented data indicating that physiological effects of a thorough active warm-up may be of substantial benefit to athletic performance. They studied endurance-trained men during a 4-min maximum aerobic treadmill run (100% $\dot{V}O_2$ max) after active or passive warm-up or rest. When preceded by active warm-up oxygen uptake was higher, lactate concentration was lower, and blood pH was higher than when preceded by passive warm-up or rest. The difference in total oxygen uptake during the run following active and passive warm-up was 0.8 litres. However, no significant difference in minute volume of expired air or respiratory quotient was found (table 3).

Passive Warm-Up

The use of hot showers prior to competition in order to improve the performance has been utilized particularly by swimmers. Following 8-min hot showers, Carlile [14] observed faster 40- and 220-yard swim times. However, in a similar study De Vries [19] did not observe improved 100-yard swim times following a 6-min hot shower. Unfortunately, treatment conditions were not randomized in either investigation and this may have influenced the results.

In addition to hot showers De Vries [19] also compared massage (passive warming up) with active warm-up using calisthenics and swimming. When swimming was used as a warm-up, 100-yard swimming times improved. Calisthenics improved the results with both breast-stroke and butterfly swimming. However, neither hot showers not massage had any effect on swim times.

Massage has also been tested on runners. Karpovich and Hale [18] observed slower 440-yard (402-meter) times following massage when compared with no warm-up at all.

Warm-Up with Repetitive Movements

Repetitive movements or movement series seem to improve performance. The warm-up effect caused by repetition has been investigated by Hipple [70], Rochelle et al. [71], Singer and Beaver [72], and Swegan et al. [73]. In general, movements performed at the beginning or at the end of a movement series are slower and less correct than those in between. However, Hipple [70] used 50-yard runs repeated five times at 5-min intervals and observed slower times towards the end of the test series, apparently due to fatigue.

The effect of warm-up on fast and sudden performances has also been investigated using both in long and high jumping. When subjects completed 90 or more vertical jumps following isometric stretching, isotonic exercise (stationary running) or a combination (knee bends) their performances improved compared with no preliminary exercise [74, 75]. Stationary running produced the greatest improvement (7.8%). The improvement appeared to be proportional to the amount of warm-up. Apparently, such results are not universal because Pyke [68] found improvement in the long jump following warm-up.

Some data indicate that using a heavier ball or javelin for warm-up can improve performance in competitions, when normal weight equipment is used (overload warm-up). Under field conditions, Bramford [76] found that after specific warm-up with a heavy 1,000-gram javelin 2 throwers improved their best training distances with a regulation weight 800 g javelin. It is unclear whether the underlying explanation for this result is neurophysiological or psychological.

Practical Applications in Various Sports

Sprints and Hurdles

Warm-up for sprints/hurdles consists of general warm-up, specific warm-up and mental training, which is particularly important in the hurdles. The explosive and rapid performance increases the risk of injury, which is why general warm-up must be very thorough. Specific warm-up should create a state of relaxation and vigour so that an explosive and concentrated performance can occur.

The sprinter usually begins his warm-up with slow sprint-like dashes and stretching. The purpose of this is to increase the circulation and temperature of the functioning muscles, eliminating stiffness and minimizing the risk of muscular injuries. Sprinters should warm-up for a relatively long time (up to 2 h). Towards the end of this process, specific warm-up is used to achieve the best possible physiological and psychological state of readiness.

Massage may be part of the warm-up for sprinters, and it is best included in the stage of general warm-up. The purpose of massage is to relax the muscles, not to make them flacid. Massage must be performed on the muscles of both the lower limbs and the back. Stretching and relaxation with or without massage may help to relieve excessive tension.

In specific warm-up, the runner seeks the right stride frequency and practices starting, running both the curves and the straight sections, tripping and accelerating. Short dashes (30–80 m) should be performed at 60–80% of maximal intensity. These should be repeated in series of 2–6 with 2–6 min of recovery. The dashes in general warm-up must not be at top speed. Mental training should occur toward the end of the warm-up process.

Warm-up can be stopped 20–30 min before the start, but it is very important to keep moving as much as possible during the interval between the warm-up and the contest. This prevents body temperature to decrease.

The warm-up for sprinters and hurdlers is a more 'exact' process than for skiers and endurance runners, and it may therefore be wise to carry it out completely under the supervision of the coach or in accordance with his instructions. Notable accelerative and muscular forces are used in sprints which may bring about musculoskeletal injuries after inadequate warm-up. Good coordination is important in the hurdles, and the ways to achieve this coordination include relaxed running of the hurdles and running by lifting up the knees.

Endurance Running

A general warm-up of 30–40 min can be considered sufficient in endurance running, although some long-distance runners may warm-up for even twice this time. However, a warm-up of an hour or more consumes quite a lot of the energy that is needed in the actual race. According to some findings, endurance runners would benefit from the relatively short, but high-intensity general warm-up.

The general warm-up of endurance runners should include running 50–400 m at different speeds. These runs are usually 100–200 m long, and are repeated 2–6 times after recovery periods. The length of the pauses between the repeated runs can vary substantially. Endurance runners take much longer warm-up runs than do sprinters, in order to become accustomed to the actual competitive speed. Massage can also be used during the initial stage of the general warm-up.

As running competitions generally take place in warm conditions, transitional warm-up is usually unneccessary. Runners therefore try to keep warm-up until 2–4 min before the start, if possible. In a warm environment the physiological effects of warm-up are maintained well for this short period. In colder weather the effect of warm-up can be maintained with warm clothing.

Specific warm-up is not as important in endurance running as it is in sports requiring skill and technique. The parts of specific warm-up, such as trying out the competitive speed, concentration, mental preparation and tactics, should be included in the general warm-up. Before the start, both calisthenics and stretching are used to increase muscular circulation in the lower limbs.

Throwing Events

For throwers the general warm-up should last about 10 min and is designed to improve specific warm-up by increasing body temperature and muscle bloodflow. Specific warm-up is very important for it allows the thrower to get kinesthetic sense of the correct movement or series of movements and to avoid injuries. Specific warm-up includes movements that are as close as possible to the actual competitive performance. The intensity of these movements should increase gradually. It is not wise, however, to aim at maximal throwing performances during warm-up, as they tend to impair mental readiness. Submaximal performances give the thrower a feeling of being able to improve. Specific warm-up should last for 10–20 min, including 5 min of special calisthenics with the throwing object, to get the feel of it. After this, throwing movements or throws with the object are made 3–5 times, in order to find the rhythm of movement. A few throws are made at 70–90% of maximal intensity, followed by a few short runs. A few examples of specific warm-up for putting the shot and throwing the discus and the javelin are given below. The movements mentioned can be repeated 2–4 times.

For shot putting, the shot is pushed strongly with the fingers from one hand into the other, with the hands in front of the body. Next, the shot is passed around the body, pushed high from a squatting position, thrown backwards over the head and pushed with both hands from chest height in a medium squatting position. A standing throw is simulated without the shot. Standing throws with the shot are made at 60% of maximal intensity. The whole throwing performance is simulated with and without the shot at 70–80% of maximal intensity. Short dashes of 15–20 m are run on the throwing ground.

In discus throwing, standing throws without the discus are simulated and standing throws with the discus are made at 60% of maximal intensity. Successive turning jumps are made along a straight line. The whole throwing performance is simulated with and without the discus at 70–80% of maximal intensity. Short dashes of 15–20 m are run.

The javelin is turned around the head with extended arms. In a slight straddle, the javelin is held up with extended arms and the body is bent forward. In a straddle, the upper part of the body is bent 90° and turned right and left with the javelin. The feet are kept parallel, with the knees slightly bent. Standing throws are simulated without the javelin. The javelin is thrown after two walking steps with the arm extended in the initial position. The whole trowing performance is made at 70–80% of maximal intensity. Dashes of 15–20 m are run.

Wrestling

For wrestlers, warm-up before training usually includes calisthenics conducted and supervised by the coach. Especially in the case of young wrestlers, the pretraining warm-up should last for 20–30% of the time spent in training. Careful preparation is necessary in wrestling to avoid tendon and muscle injuries, which otherwise occur quite frequently.

Wrestling requires speed, endurance, strength, technical skill, quick perception, and agility. Initially, the warm-up should be as general as possible. As the warm-up proceeds the movements should become more specific. For young wrestlers, warm-up should emphasize agility and suppleness, and their program should thus include quite difficult calisthenic movements, e.g. somersaults. In the adult, these movements can be replaced with muscle condition or technical training.

Warm-up should be slightly different under training camp conditions from what it is at home, because in the camp there are frequent encounters with training partners. Long and light general warm-up (e.g. ball games) is recommended, because it does not consume the energy resources needed for the actual performances and it keeps up the mental vigour, which tends to disappear during a long training camp. During camps it is also possible for the coaches to teach the wrestlers the best warmup techniques and to correct obvious mistakes.

On the day of the contest, general warm-up should begin in the morning, using running and easy wrestling. The purpose of this is to practise movement routines and to relieve tension. This initial warm-up increases body temperature and activates the oxygen transport and metabolic systems. It should therefore be relatively short in duration, i.e. about 20 min, in order to conserve energy, as making weight may have been a hard effort. After that the wrestler may bathe, watch the others wrestle, do some stretching movements and perhaps have a light massage. Between this and the final warm-up he may observe his future opponent and plan strategy.

The final preparation for the contest is relatively short, i.e. 10–15 min, consisting of repetition of right movements, light massage and shaking. At the stage of massage and shaking, which is strength saving, mainly passive warm-up, a flacid wrestler can be envigorated and a tense wrestler calmed down. The wrestler must have the fighting spirit right from the beginning, and this spirit should be created at the final stage of warm-up.

Massage or passive warm-up just before a contest may suit some but not all wrestlers. Intensive and thorough massage probably makes the muscles flaccid. To avoid this the massage should be performed quickly, with short and sharp motions. The final stage of warm-up should concentrate on increasing speed, agility and controlled aggression.

Archery

Initial warm-up in archery has both psychological and physiological goals. Its purpose is to create sufficient alertness and to relieve tension

(tension released as physical activity) as well as to increase muscular circulation and metabolism. However, in archery these physiological conditions are not critical, and thus the warm-up need not be lengthy. An initial warm-up of 10 min should be sufficient, and it can be performed walking or running.

After this initial warm-up, the muscles of the back, the shoulders and the upper limbs should be stretched. This will activate the muscles needed in archery, relieve muscular tension, and improve nerve-muscle coordination. For specific warm-up, a few arrows can be discharged at a short distance towards an empty background. This stage of warm-up takes about 5 min. After this, ordinary training can be begun. Before a contest, 10–15 min should be reserved for relaxation and mental training, where details are gone over and a mental balance is sought. The initial warm-up and stretching help the archer to concentrate and to achieve a feeling of confidence.

Arousal and muscular tension increase during a contest, and therefore it may be useful to utilize passive warm-up methods, e.g. massage, between the periods of competition.

Although, from the physiological point of view, initial warm-up does not seem to be of great significance in archery as it is in other sports, it has been found to diminish the risk of strain injuries due to the discharging movements, and to have a favourable effect on performance. During archery contests, cool down is equally important as warm-up, because it helps to maintain a suitable level of alertness for the following day of competition.

Cross-Country Skiing

In cross-country skiing, as in all outdoor winter sports, thorough general warm-up is very important. The intensity and duration of warm-up however, depend somewhat on the temperature. In cold environments, as in the Nordic countries, warm-up may take a few hours. In Central European countries, where the daytime temperature may be relatively high (even in winter), an excessively long warm-up may be counterproductive.

The primary goal of general warm-up in skiing is to elevate body temperature. The problem is keeping the body temperature high and avoiding getting cold. This can be achieved by adding clothing after the warm-up.

The general warm-up of a skier usually includes both skiing and running. It is necessary to include some running in the warm-up because the faster pace of running helps to adapt to the rhythm of skiing.

General warm-up may consist of running for 1–2 km with some

low-intensity dashes of 10–100 m and some calisthenic movements with stretching. Next, some higher intensity dashes should be performed, e.g. 4–5 times 100–200 m, followed by a final jog of about 5 min. The general warm-up is usually sufficient when the skier begins to sweat. The increased body temperature must be maintained during the specific warm-up.

With the new skiing techniques (skating), specific warm-up has become even more important. Specific warm-up can be accomplished by skiing rapid dashes (uphill and downhill), trying to find the optimal speed and technique. The skating technique places greater strain on the muscles of the arms, the back, the buttocks and the thighs when compared to the diagonal technique. Hence, the specific training for the skating technique includes movements which enhance circulation and activate muscles in these areas. The skating technique and the diagonal technique differ significantly from each other, and the specific warm-up for the skating technique should be technically similar to that for ice skating (see below).

Skating

Before competition the warm-up should begin with jogging, calisthenics and stretching. Once on the ice the first few rounds should be skated slowly, getting the muscles used to skating. Thereafter, intensity is increased by skating a few near maximal accelerations. Finally, one should practice starting.

After this warm-up, it is necessary to sharpen the skates and take care of the outfit. During this time it is necessary to stay warm and to concentrate on the upcoming competition. Some skaters may use massage during this period. Once back on the ice, movements involved in the coordination of skating are performed.

Skaters usually compete several times a day, which makes interval warm-up necessary. The purpose of interval warm-up is to recover from the preceding competition and to prepare for the following one. Lactic acid is best eliminated when exercise intensity is about 60% of $\dot{V}O_2$ max.

Before the second skating competition, the warm-up procedure should be similar to that mentioned above for the first competition. If the skating distance is long, the warm-up must be prolonged, but at a lower intensity than before shorter distance events. This warm-up should enhance the functioning of the respiratory and circulatory systems as well as activating the muscles to be used in skating.

With regular training sessions interval warm-up is unneccessary. Otherwise the warm-up before training is similar to that before a competition.

Warm-up before training is necessary, because the objectives of training may otherwise remain unattained. Warm-up should not be conceptually confused with training. It is not part of a training but rather a separate stage necessary in the preparation of the skater for training.

Mental training can also be useful in preparing a skater for competition. The skating of the straights and curves, for example, can be imagined. During warm-up a skater should concentrate on the technical and tactical details of the performance and analyze the opponent's strengths and weaknesses.

Skating is a winter sport and therefore environmental temperature must be taken into account when planning the warm up. The colder the weather, the more thorough the warm-up must be. The increased body temperature achieved by means of warm-up is quickly lost, unless clothing is sufficient. If the clothing is inadequate it is not possible to attain the benefits of warm-up no matter how well it is designed or realized.

Ice Hockey

In ice hockey, warm-up is used as the initial stage of training both off and on the ice and as a part of the preparation for a match. During the period of basic conditioning in the summer months, the training is preceded by warm-up with jogging and active and passive stretching movements. Once organized training begins it is critical to continue to use warm-up, because it is the most effective way of preventing strains of the back and lower limb muscles. In ice training the heavy outfit makes some warm-up movements difficult or even impossible. Therefore, most of the warm-up should be performed before going onto the ice (e.g. jogging, doing calisthenics and stretching in the corridor or outdoors). When the training or the match take place outdoors in winter temperatures, the warm-up must be started by gradually increasing the intensity before beginning the training or the match.

Prior to a match or training session warm-up may be supervised by the coach in the locker room. The movements must be performed rapidly, e.g. as jumps and stationary running with increasing intensity. The warm-up should be designed to prepare the athletes both physiologically and psychologically for the competition.

Frequently prior to matches ice time is too short for adequate warm-up. In this case, general warm-up to increase metabolism and to elevate the body temperature can be accomplished by jogging and playing different ball games. This can be followed by locker room warm-up of higher intensity, which includes jumps and different calisthenic movements. The final warm-up of 20 min should take place on the ice just before the beginning of the match. If time is short, the elevation of body temperature must be achieved with running and various locker room activities.

Under tournament conditions the significance of warm-up increases. Ice hockey requires speed, endurance, strength, technical skill, quick perception and cooperation. Light initial warm-up can be used to elevate the body temperature and to increase physiological readiness. Also, by increasing the intensity at the final stage of the warm-up, it is possible to relieve excessive tension and anxiety.

Final preparations for the game is made by skating, stickhandling and reviewing strategy. At this stage individual players can motivate each other by shouting instructions, such as: skate, attack, check, and fight!

Warm-Up and Injury

The role of warm-up in preventing injuries has been emphasized frequently. The temperature of a resting muscle is slightly lower than deep body temperature, and therefore muscular elasticity may be enhanced by increasing muscle temperature [77]. This might explain why warm-up enhances performance.

In a group of schoolchildren Mathews and Snyder [66] studied effects of warm-up on the frequency of muscular injuries during 400-yard runs at maximum speed. No injuries occurred under either condition but a conclusion from these data is difficult because subjects were not elite runners (400 yard time = 61.4–90.5 s) and the number studied was relatively small (n = 50). Similarly, no muscular injuries were observed by Rochelle et al. [71] or Ryan and Almann [78] who studied subjects (n = 46) throwing a soft ball.

Koppel [79] believes that proper warm-up is not only important in improving physical performance, but also in prevention of autogenous injuries. He has described some fatal cases associated with exercise which may have been avoided if adequate warm-up had occurred. According to Barnard et al. [80, 91], warm-up can also prevent some electrocardiogram abnormalities (ST segment depression) that are sometimes seen in healthy persons at the beginning of fast running performances.

Cool Down

Methods of Cool Down
The purpose of cool down is to facilitate recovery following a maximal competitive performance. Just as warm-up is a step between rest and maximal performance which improves the performance capacity, cool down is a step from maximal performance to rest which facilitates recovery. Although cool down is at least as complex as warm-up, it has received much less attention.

Cool down makes it possible to attain a physiological balance more quickly after competition. Maximal performances can result in the formation of lactic acid, which should be eliminated as soon as possible or subsequent performance will be adversely affected. Active cool down has been found to eliminate lactic acid much more quickly than rest [82]. The oxygen debt is also compensated for more quickly. Breathing oxygen, however, has not been shown to accelerate the elimination of lactic acid [82]. Cool down helps to relieve muscular tension after maximal strain. The muscles attain their resting length sooner, and the prolonged pains due to muscular tension may be prevented.

Cool down is also important for reaching an emotional balance after the possible disappointment of a poor performance. In situations where the next competition follows soon afterwards, it is even possible to begin to prepare for it during the cool down from the initial performance. An athlete's emotions can be highly agitated before and during the competition and although the end of the performance alleviates the physical stress, emotional turmoil may continue for a long time. An athlete's thoughts (positive or negative) may keep returning to the competition and cool down can help one to analyze the causes of success or failure. The coach may assist in this situation. As an observer, his opinion regarding the performance may help the athlete return to reality. Failure in a competition may best be addressed at this time because feedback is most beneficial if given soon after the performance. It is good to remember that mental recovery is a prerequisite for successful physical recovery.

Practical Applications

In a similar manner to warm-up, cool down can be carried out either actively or passively. Today one sees most top athletes employ some planned cool down after the competition. Usually, this involves stretching movements and moving about actively.

Relaxed stretching and shaking of the muscles are an essential part of active cool down. The goal is to make the muscles return to their resting length, to improve their circulation and to prevent the formation of muscular hardenings. After strenuous training, muscle stretching should be performed 2–3 h later. At that time the stretching of the muscles is less uncomfortable than it might be immediately after the training.

As mentioned above, it can be useful to use the cool down period to analyze the past performance part by part and to consider the possible ways of improving it. This retrospective analysis frequently helps the athlete to relax and view the performance more objectively. It also permits one to begin to plan for future competitions which may occur quite soon. This is especially true in tournament competition or in sports with frequent competitive events.

Traditionally passive procedures have been of more marked significance in cool down than in warm-up. Passive cool down (e.g. massage, stretching, sauna and warm showers) does not, however, compensate for neglected active cool down.

Conclusion

Warm-up and cool down have obvious physiological and psychological effects which can improve physical performance capacity and/or facilitate recovery. Although it is difficult to imagine an athlete who would not warm-up before a competition and would not feel it to be beneficial, several investigators of the physiological and psychological effects of warm-up have obtained contradictory results concerning the benefits of warm-up on performance. However, definitive information is difficult to obtain because the complexity of the warm-up phenomenon makes it nearly impossible to simulate in the laboratory, or even to standardize in the field.

Investigations have been made on groups of schoolchildren or students of physical education, whose physical performance capacity is not similar to that of top athletes. Many studies have been on very small samples, some consisting of only 2–3 subjects. Moreover, the content, duration and intensity of warm-up have varied dramatically from almost no activity (light bending and straightening of the knees) to very intense exercise (pedalling a bicycle ergometer, jogging or sprint-like dashes). It seems that some studies have not considered the disadvantages of inadequate warm-up. It appears that the amount of activity needed for warm-up and cool down largely depend on the individual and on the weather conditions.

There is some agreement concerning the physiological effects of warm-up. For example, during general warm-up, the body temperature rises, which significantly improves the physical performance capacity. Activation of the respiration and the circulation improves muscular blood flow and oxygen uptake. Oxygen is better released from hemoglobin and myoglobin, which further improves oxygen uptake in the tissues. Muscle viscosity decreases, which results in an improvement of muscular mechanical efficiency. The velocity of nerve impulses and the sensitivity of nervous receptors also increase. The risk of injuries and cardiovascular complications decrease. All these factors significantly improve the performance capacity.

During warm-up the athlete can impose his mental readiness by concentrating on the imminent competition. Warm-up time is also useful for planning strategy and controlling arousal levels. Specific warm-up can improve an individual's nerve-muscle coordination and kinesthetic sense, and in addition to provide a chance for imaginative training.

The duration and intensity of warm-up are fundamental questions, which depend largely on the type of sport in question, the individual, and the environmental conditions. In general, active warm-up and cool down are more beneficial than passive.

In practice, athletes should warm-up for 1–2 h, varying the intensity from 40 to 100% of the maximum. The average intensity of warm-up is about 60% of the maximum. Signs of sweating are a good indicator of the effectiveness of the warm-up. The elevation of body temperature achieved by warm-up is retained for 20–30 min, if the individual keeps active or if appropriate clothing is worn.

Cool down can help relieve the physical and psychic tensions created by the competition. Active cool down helps to facilitate physiological recovery, eliminate lactic acid and return the muscles to their resting length. Cool down also provides an opportunity to evaluate and analyze the performance.

Warm-up seems to be most beneficial in sports with require strength, speed, endurance and skill. It is obvious that warm-up is more effective, the more fully the athlete believes in its effects.

References

1 Caralis DG, Edwards L, Davis PJ: Serum total and free thyroxine and triiodothyronine during dynamic muscular exercise in man. Am J Physiol 1977;233:E115–E118.
2 Jürgensen P: Die Körperwärme des gesunden Menschen. Leipzig, 1873, p 47.
3 Pembrey MS, Nicol BA: Observations upon the deep and surface temperature of the human body. J Physiol 1898;23:386.
4 Christensen EH: Beiträge zur Physiologie schwerer körperlicher Arbeit. Arbeitsphysiologie 1931;4:154.
5 Ruosteenoja R: Studies on circulatory, respiratory and thermal adaption during heavy exercise. Acta Physiol Scand 1954;31:256–261.
6 Harrison MH, Edwards RJ, Leitch DR: Effect of exercise and thermal stress on plasma volume. J Appl Physiol 1975;39:926.
7 Zuntz N, Schumburg J: In: Studien zu einer Physiologie des Marsches. Berlin, Verlag von August Hirschwald, 1901, pp 315–316.
8 Zuntz N, Loewy A, Muller F, Caspari W: In: Hönhenklima und Bergwanderungen. Berlin, 1906, p 60.
9 Hill AV: Living machinery; In: Six Lectures Delivered at the Royal Institution. London, Bell, 1945, pp 1–42.
10 Simonson EN, Teslenko J, Gorkin M: Einfluss von Übungen auf die Leistung beim 100 m Lauf. Arbeitsphysiologie 1936;9:152.
11 Nielsen M: Die Regulation der Körpertemperatur bei Muskelarbeit. Scand Arch Physiol 1938;79:193–229.
12 Asmussen E, Böje O: Body temperature and capacity for work. Acta Physiol Scand 1945;10:1–21.
13 Muido L: The influence of body temperature on performance in swimming Acta Physiol Scand 1946;12:102.

14   Carlile F: Effect of preliminary passive warming on swimming performance. Res Q Am
      Assoc Health Phys Educ 1956;27:143–151.

15   Kelitman N, Titelbaum S, Feiveson P: The effect of body temperature on reaction
      time. Am J Physiol 1938;121:495–501.

16   Du Bois EF: The basal metabolism in fever. J Am Med Assoc 1921;77:352.

17   Nielsen B: Thermoregulation in rest and exercise. Acta Physiol Scand 1969;(suppl
      323):63–65.

18   Karpovitch PV, Hale CJ: Effect of warming-up upon physical performance. JAMA
      1956;162:1117–1119.

19   De Vries HA: Effects of various warm-up procedures on 100-yard times of competitive
      swimmers. Res Q Am Assoc Health Phys Educ 1959;30:11–20.

20   Grucza R, Lecroart JL, Hauser JJ, Houdas Y: Dynamics of sweating in men and
      women during passive heating. Eur J Appl Physiol 1985;54:309–314.

21   Grucza R, Hänninen O: Importance of dynamics of sweating in men during exercise;
      Acta Physiol Pol 1990;41:65–75.

22   Chwalbinska-Moneta J, Hänninen O: Effect of active warming-up on thermoregula-
      tory, circulatory, and metabolic responses to incremental exercise in endurance-trained
      athletes. Int J Sports Med 1989;10:25–29.

23   Danfort WH: Activation of glycolytic pathway in muscle; in Chance B, Estabrook
      RW, Williamson JR (eds): Control of Energy Metabolism. New York, Academic
      Press, 1965, pp 287–297.

24   Karlson J, Hulten B, Sjödin B: Substrate activation and product inhibition of LDH
      activity in human skeletal muscle. Acta Physiol Scand 1974;92:21–26.

25   Margaria R, Edwards HT, Dill DB: The possible mechanism of contraction and
      paying the oxygen dept and the role of lactic acid in muscular contraction. Am J
      Physiol 1933;106:689–714.

26   Margaria R, Geretelli P, di Prampero PE, Massari C, Torelli G: Kinetics and mecha-
      nism of oxygen dept contraction in man. J Appl Physiol 1963;18:371–377.

27   Cobb LA, Johnson WP: Hemodynamic relationship of anaerobic metabolism and
      plasma free fatty acids during prolonged strenuous exercise in trained and untrained
      subjects. J Clin Invest 1963;42:800–809.

28   Williams CG, Wyndham CH, Kok R, von Rahden MJE: Effect of training on
      maximum oxygen intake and on anaerobic metabolism in man. Int Z Angew Physiol
      1967;24:18.

29   Keul J: Energy metabolism during submaximal exercise. XXVII Int Congr Physiologi-
      cal Sciences. Paris, July, 1977, Abstr, vol XII, p 724.

30   Karvonen J: Warming-up and its physiological effects. Acta Univ Ouluensis Pharm
      Physiol 1978;30:1–50.

31   Yamaguchi A: Study on the effects of warm-up on trained and untrained subjects.
      Proc Dep Phys Educ Univ Tokyo 1967;4:9–14.

32   Saltin B: Aerobic work capacity and circulation at exercise in man. Acta Physiol Scand
      1964;(suppl 230):7–10.

33   Hickson RC, Bomze HA, Holloszy JO: Faster adjustment of O_2 uptake to the energy
      requirement of exercise in the trained state. J Appl Physiol 1978;44:877–881.

34   Ingjer F, Strömme SB: Effects of active, passive or no warm-up on the physiological
      response to heavy exercise. Eur J Appl Physiol 1979;40:273–282.

35   Wigertz O: Dynamics of respiratory and circulatory adaption to muscular exercise in
      man. Acta Physiol Scand 1971;(suppl 363).

36   Paulev PE: Respiratory and cardiac responses to exercise in man. J Appl Physiol
      1971;30:165–172.

37   Ekelund LC: Circulatory and respiratory adaption during prolonged exercise in the supine position. Acta Physiol Scand 1966;68:388–390.

38   Ekelund LC: Circulatory and respiratory adaption during prolonged exercise of moderate intensity in the sitting position. Acta Physiol Scand 1967;69:332–335.

39   Barcroft J, King WOR: The effect of temperature on the dissociation curve of blood. J Physiol 1909;39:374.

40   Liesen H, Hollmann W, Fotescu MD, Mathur DN: Lungenfunktion, Atmung und Stoffwechsel im Sport; in Hollmann W (ed): Zentrale Themen der Sport-medizin. Berlin, Springer, 1972, p 70.

41   Stegemann J: In: Leistungsphysiologie. Stuttgart, Thieme, 1977, p 104.

42   Faulkner JA, Brewer GJ, Eaton JW: Red cell metabolism and function; In Brewer G (ed): Adaption of the Red Cells to Muscular Exercise. New York, Plenum Press, 1970, pp 213–229.

43   Brundin T: Temperature of mixed venous blood during exercise. Scand J Clin Lab Invest 1975;35:539–543.

44   Ramsey JD, Ayoub M, Dudek R, Edgar H: Heart rate recovery during a college basketball game. Res Q Am Assoc Health Phys Educ 1970;41:528.

45   Arnold A: In: Lehrbuch der Sportmedizin. Leipzig, Johann Ambrosius Barth Verlag, 1960, pp 170–171.

46   Sjöstrand Å: Die Schlagfrequenz des Herzens während und nach der Leistung; In Arnold A (ed): Lehrbuch der Sportmedizin. Leipzig, Johann Ambrosius Barth Verlag, 1960, p 30.

47   Klint F, Nitschke M: Radiotelemetrische Herzstrom-Kurvenregistrierungen während eines schulsportlichen Übungszyklus. Dt Gesundheitsw 1971;26:64–70.

48   Knowlton RG, Miks DS, Sawka MN: Metabolic responses of untrained individuals to warm-up. Eur J Appl Physiol 1978;40:1–5.

49   De Bryun-Prevost P: The effects of various warming-up intensities and duration upon some physiological variables during an exercise corresponding to the WC170. Eur J Appl Physiol 1980;113:93–100.

50   Clasing D, Vogler G, Burchardt W, Klaus EJ: Herzfrequenz und psychische Anspannung beim Segelfliegen. Med Welt 1971;19:808–810.

51   Christian P, Spohr U: Fortlaufende, simultane Kreislaufmessungen während biographischer Interviews mit telemetrischen Methoden. Psychosom Med 1970;16:1–4.

52   Brundin T, Cernigliaro C: The effect of physical training on the sympathoadrenal response to exercise. Scand J Clin Lab Invest 1975;35:525–530.

53   Pavlik G: Lisämunuaisten erittämien hormoonien merkitys harjoittelussa; In: Urheilulääketieteen jatkoseminaari (SVUL). Vierumäki, 1976, pp 5–10.

54   Meythaler F: Die Regulation des Kohlenhydratstoffwechsels bei Sport. Klin Wochenschr 1937;27:951.

55   Malarecki J: In Frost J (ed): Psychological Concepts Applied to Physical Education and Coaching. New York, Addison Wesley, 1971, pp 201–206.

56   Puni AC: Psychological Preparation for Sport Contests. Moscow, Figkultura i Sport, 1969, p 8.

57   Blanz F: Keskittymistapahtuma; In Blanz F, Kalliokoski A, Suonperä M, Tomperi K (eds): Urheiluvalmennuksen psykologiaa. Helsinki, Suomen Valtakunnan Urheiluliitto ry, 1973, pp 82–86.

58   Schmidt P: Frustration und Vorstartperiode. Schweiz Z Sportmed 1975;23:93.

59   Smith JL, Bozymowski MF: Effect of altitude toward warm-up on motor performance. Res Q Am Assoc Health Phys Educ 1965;36:78–83.

60   Massey BH, Johnson WR, Kramer GF: Effect of warm-up exercise upon muscular

performance using hypnosis to control the physiological variable. Res Q Am Assoc Health Phys Educ 1961;32:63.

61 Yerker-Dodson V: In Fisher AC (ed): Psychology of Sport. Palo Alto, Mayfield, 1976, p 119.

62 Oxendine A: In Fischer AC (ed): Psychology of Sport. Palo Alto, Mayfield, 1976, p 126.

63 Corcoran D: Personality and the inverted-U relation. Br J Psychol 1965;56:267–273.

64 Högberg P, Ljunggren O: Uppvärmningens inverkan på löpprestationerna. Svensk Idrott 1947;40:668–671.

65 Blank LB: Effects of warm-up on speed. Athletic J 1955;35:10–45.

66 Mathews DK, Snyder HA: Effect of warm-up on the 440 yard dash. Res Q Am Assoc Health Phys Educ 1959;30:446–450.

67 Grodjinowski A, Magel JR: Effect of warm-up on running performance. Res Q Am Assoc Health Phys Educ 1970;41:116–118.

68 Pyke FS: The effect of preliminary activity on maximal motor performance. Re Q Am Assoc Health Phys Educ 1968;39:1069.

69 Masterovoj LI: Die zweckmässige Intensität der Aufwärmung. Theor Praxis Körperkultur 1969:539.

70 Hipple JE: Warm-up and fatigue in junior high school sprinters. Res Q Am Assoc Health Phys Educ 1955;26:246–247.

71 Rochelle RH, Skubic V, Michael ED: Performance as affected by incentive and preliminary warm-up. Res Q Am Assoc Health Phys Educ 1960;31:499–503.

72 Singer NR, Beaver R: Bowling and the warm-up effect. Res Q Am Assoc Health Phys Educ 1969;40:372–375.

73 Swegan DB, Yankosky TG, Williams Jr III: Effect of repetition upon speed of preferred-arm extension. Res Q Am Assoc Health Phys Educ 1958;29:74.

74 Pacheco BA: Improvement in jumping performance due to preliminary exercise. Res Q Am Assoc Health Phys Educ 1957;28:55–63.

75 Pacheco BA: Effectiveness of warm-up exercise in junior high school girls. Res Q Am Assoc Health Phys Educ 1959;30:202–213.

76 Bramford M: The value of warm up. Athletics Coach 1985;19:13.

77 Nöcker J: In: Physiologie der Leibesübungen. Stuttgart, Ferdinand Enke, 1971, pp 57–58.

78 Ryan AJ, Almann FL Jr: In: Sportsmedicine. New York, Academic Press, 1974, pp 138, 481–482, 613.

79 Kopell, HP: The warm-up and autogeneous injury. NY State J Med 1962;62:3255–3258.

80 Barnard RJ, Gardner GW, Diaco NV, McAlpin RN, Kattus AA: Cardiovascular responses to sudden strenuous exercise-heart rate, blood pressure and ECG. J Appl Physiol 1973;34:833–837.

81 Barnard RJ, McAlpin R, Kattus AA, Buckberg GD: Ischemic response to sudden strenuous exercise in healthy men. Circulation 1973;158:936–942.

82 Weltman A, Stamford BA, Moffatt RJ, Katch VL: Exercise recovery, lactate removal, and subsequent high intensity exercise performance. Res Q Am Assoc Health Phys Educ 1977;48:789–791.

Dr. Juha Karvonen, National Agency for Welfare and Health, P.O. Box 220, SF-00531 Helsinki (Finland)

Karvonen J, Lemon PWR, Iliev I (eds): Medicine in Sports Training and Coaching.
Med Sport Sci. Basel, Karger, 1992, vol 35, pp 215–234

Mental Training

Seppo E. Iso-Ahola

College of Health and Human Performance, University of Maryland,
College Park, Md., USA

Contents

Introduction

Exceptional athletic performance is no longer a simple matter of physical ability and training. It is safe to say that regardless of sports, superior athletes are mentally tougher than less superior athletes. In some sports, mental performance is more important than in others, but there is no athletic activity in which performance would not be enhanced by mental strength. For an example, consider golf. Just about all professional golfers on the PGA tour hit the ball 270 yards and straight off the tee; they all hit their irons crisply and putt with splendid touch. So, their physical and technical skills are quite equal. What then separates the winner from the loser? It is the winner's self-confidence, his or her determination or 'willpower', skill to concentrate and manage anxiety. In short, it is 'athletic intelligence' or a person's overall psychological capacity or aptitude to perform in mentally demanding and stressful competitive situations [1].

Although there may be some variation in these factors of athletic intelligence between individual sports (e.g. long-distance running vs. rifle-shooting), they nevertheless are important to successful performers in all sports. In team sports, psychological characteristics also play an important role, but interpersonal factors take on added significance. Of these, team motivation, spirit and cohesiveness are perhaps the most significant.

A question, then, is how to acquire mental toughness to become a winner. It is obvious that some individuals are physiologically or biologically better off in this regard than others. But much more is involved here than biological differences between individuals. To become a winner is largely a matter of social learning. Athletes learn from opponents, teachers, coaches and sport psychologists the psychological characteristics and tools needed to become winners. They learn that mental training is as important as physical training if one is to succeed in his or her sports.

What Is Mental Training?

Sport psychologists do not give a uniform definition for mental training. The term has been used rather loosely and in a global sense to refer to various aspects of training focused on cognitive and affective functioning of an athlete. Williams [2] equates it with psychological skills training, while Mahoney [3] divides it into two types: last-minute preparations before performance and mental rehearsal or practice. To Kirschenbaum [4], mental training is self-regulation of sport performance. In the midst of these different approaches, one can find one common thread to mental training: skill-training for performance enhancement. Skills, in turn, refer to a host of acquired tendencies to motivate oneself, boost self-confidence, manage anxiety and stress, concentrate better, physically relax through different techniques, and mentally rehearse performance via such techniques as internal and external imagery. In general, mental practice functions to assist the performer in psychologically preparing for the skill to be performed [5].

If the term 'mental training' is used too loosely, it would have to include all psychological methods coaches use to improve team performance, such as psyching up pep-talks. However, most sport psychologists would probably agree that such a definition of the term is too general and consequently misleading. Most appropriately, the term should be used to refer to individual training that strives systematically and purposefully to improve an athlete's cognitive (e.g. thinking, planning and concentration) and affective (e.g. feelings and fears) skills needed in sport performance. Although such training can occur in group sessions and with the help of outside agents (e.g. sport psychologists), it is ultimately the individual athlete who is doing the training for himself or herself. In this sense, then, mental training is indeed self-regulation. It largely revolves around self-control, be it control over one's emotions, fears and anxieties, or internal locus of control, a belief that one can and will succeed and win.

A major goal of mental training is achievement of the three Cs of mental performance: *control, challenge and commitment*. An athlete has to have commitment to his or her sport. It means that an athlete must have an ambition to be a world-class performer on the one hand and willingness to go through all the physical and technical training required to succeed at that level on the other. An athlete must have a sense of control over his or her emotions, cognitions, and behaviors. He or she must develop a sense of belief in oneself and personal abilities and that everything is possible through effort and hard work. An athlete who is in control over his/her emotions is able to manage anxiety and stress of competition as well as fears of success and failure. Finally, a successful athlete views difficulties, problems, hardships and opposition as a challenge rather than a threat. Underdogs who beat their opponents are such athletes. They thrive on challenging situations and opponents rather than become anxious and fearful of such events.

Mental training should lead to what Morgan [6] calls an 'iceberg profile'. When testing world-class wrestlers, runners and oarsmen, Morgan found the most successful athletes to exhibit a profile according to which they peaked at 'vigor' and scored relatively low on the following mental features: tension, depression, anger, fatigue, and confusion. High 'vigor' reflects the successful athletes' stronger determination to succeed or 'will to win'. A person with high vigor is in control over his or her emotions and behaviors and is determined to succeed. Determination also means commitment to hard work and practice required to succeed. In fact, there is evidence that top athletes develop an obsessive-compulsive style of maintaining their efforts in their sports [4]. Their compulsive behavior includes withdrawal from others, frequent self-talk, and generally living a highly structured lifestyle.

Self-Regulation

As noted above, mental training is largely a matter of self-regulation of one's cognitions, affect, physiological condition and behaviors. First and foremost, it means that the athlete takes more responsibility for his or her performance and makes commitment to behavior modification. Self-regulation also emphasizes the importance of systematically attending to feedback about one's performance, evaluating performance against specified

criteria, and working to sustain efforts despite setbacks in performance [4]. Thus, the process of self-regulation stresses the importance of :
- (a) goal-setting and positive expectations for success and performance execution;
- (b) self-monitoring relevant behaviors;
- (c) self-evaluation of performance against standards;
- (c) self-reinforcement or self-punishment depending on self-evaluation.

Goal Setting and Positive Expectations

It is well documented that goal-setting improves performance and performance outcomes [1]. Goal setting serves as a motivational vehicle to mobilize maximum effort needed to improve performance. Research suggests that athletes should be directed to set their goals personally, so that goal acceptance and commitment would be maximized. Their goals should be specific and difficult, but attainable. The overall goal should be broken down into 'proximal sub-goals', so that achievement of these subgoals would provide informative feedback about one's performance level and progress [7]. In short, personally set, specific and hard proximal subgoals with accompanying feedback are conducive to enhanced motivation and improved athletic performance. Such goals affect performance by (a) directing attention and action; (b) by mobilizing energy expenditure or effort; (c) by prolonging effort over time (persistence); and (d) by motivating the athlete to develop relevant stategies for goal attainment [8].

Goal-setting leads to positive expectations for success. Achievement of proximal subgoals gives positive feedback (knowledge of results) about one's effort and performance and thereby leads to further expectations for success. While expectancy of success is in general better than expectancy of failure, some top athletes have more of a 'fear of failure' than some of their less successful opponents. However, 'there appears to be an excessive level for everyone, and even those capable of performing well with high levels of fear of failure will eventually suffer performance disruptions if their tolerance limit is reached' [1]. Therefore, it becomes important for athletes to develop expectancies for success, and the best strategy in this regard appears to be the setting of proximal subgoals. Achievement of personal subgoals represents fulfillment of expectations of success, which in turn facilitates further setting of hard but attainable subgoals. The end result is the cycle in which success breeds success and provides conditions for 'psychological momentum' [9, 10].

Self-Monitoring, Self-Evaluation, and Self-Reinforcement

It is clear from the above discussion that goal-setting and expectations for success and performance execution are inextricably linked to one another. The discussion also suggests that athletes must self-monitor their performance and behaviors, evaluate their performance against a standard and positively reinforce or punish themselves depending on the favorableness of self-evaluation. Self-monitoring means that the athlete attends to relevant target behaviors and systematically attends to feedback about one's performance. Kirschenbaum [4] worked with a top-level golfer who had such self-monitoring problems. This athlete was sometimes too casual with his preparation before shooting. For example, he failed to take into account certain hazards on the course and the effect of windy conditions. The athlete also tended to dwell on poor previous performances such as missed 4-feet putts on earlier holes. Kirschenbaum trained the athlete to use a planning checklist before each shot, imagery before each shot, and positive self-monitoring or keeping track of successful shots. This latter technique did not allow the athlete to dwell on negative performances and forced him to postpone thinking of poor or problem shots until after the round. The athlete used a little red notebook in which he kept instructional sheets for his planning, imagery, and positive self-monitoring procedures. The book became an important and permanent part of his tournament routine during competition.

When athletes are taught to operationally define components of sport performance, they learn to self-monitor their performance. Thus, they learn to review the important components of effective performance afterwards. So, for example, bowlers do it after each frame, golfers after each shot, and long jumpers after each jump. In addition, self-monitoring should be done after the entire competition is over. Calvin Peete, one of the most successful professional golfers, said that he locks himself in his room at the end of a day after each competitive round and analyzes every shot he made during the tournament.

The self-monitoring approach is beneficial because it facilitates attentional focusing and encourages the use of self-instructions. Self-monitoring also promotes the use of highly specific, nonemotional feedback and facilitates accurate self-evaluation. As noted above, self-evaluation is best done in relation to the set goals. An athlete should evaluate his or her performance on the basis of 'knowledge of results' or feedback about performance. Such feedback is plentiful in athletic situations and has motivational effects when used in conjunction with subgoals, that is, feedback shows one's progress toward achieving goals. Such a progress report not only gives an idea whether the goal is realistic and attainable, but also how much effort is needed to achieve it within certain time limits. Knowledge of results also has motivational effects because it affects goal-setting. Research suggests that correct, positive knowledge of results significantly increases the levels of goals set [11].

It should be stressed that feedback without goals is not sufficient to improve performance. Therefore, social reinforcement (positive or negative) is effective in improving performance only to the extent that it informs an athlete about his or her performance in relation to specific goals (i.e. progress toward them) [1]. Even if specific goals have been established, feedback concerning these goals must be informative and accurate. Emotional evaluation of performance in terms of win or loss, success or failure does not promote objective self-evaluation against a standard (i.e. a goal). It does not help the athlete understand why good or poor performance occurred.

There is sufficient experimental evidence in the literature to suggest that excessive negative or positive feedback tends to erode a sense of personal control over task performance [12]. It has been shown that a coach's frequent negative and punitive remarks to his players undermine their attitudes toward the coach, themselves and playing the sport in the future [13]; such feedback also tends to impair performance itself [14]. Coaches' negative feedback leads to self-punishment on the part of individual athletes and therefore interrupts the self-regulation process. Self-reinforcement or punishment should be based upon the objective evaluation rather than on someone else's emotional interpretation of one's performance. Given the possibility of poor psychological coaching, it becomes even more important for individual athletes to set personal specific goals against which performance and self are later evaluated. An athlete who engages in the self-regulation process through self-monitoring, self-evaluation and self-reinforcement is in essence protecting himself or herself from coaches' repeated negative feedback. That is, they monitor and evaluate their performance on the basis of their personal subgoals and regulate their effort and preparation without regard to a coach's negative and punitive feedback.

Of course, everything should not be left at the mercy of self-regulation. Coaching is still an important part of athletic endeavors, but what is needed is to subject coaches to 'coach effectiveness training'. Such training emphasizes the psychological significance of a coach's work and the need to understand the psychological mechanisms underlying athletes' performance and behaviors. It emphasizes the importance of positive reinforcement and encouragement as well as technical instruction [13].

Anxiety and Stress Management

One of the main reasons why the self-regulation process is successful in improving athletic performance is because it helps in anxiety and stress management. Excessive levels of anxiety and stress are detrimental to performance and must therefore be brought under control. While many strategies for coping with performance anxiety have been introduced (e.g. training of basic relaxation skills), they all deal with the self-regulation process. So, for example, training and refinement of self-instruction skills improve athletes' coping capacities because such skills make them focus attention on task demands rather than disruptive external factors. Similarly, athletes who have been directed, taught and trained to appraise and refine personal meanings of athletic success and failure relative to personal goals are better able to cope with performance anxiety. Finally, as pointed out earlier, the entire process of self-monitoring, self-evaluation and self-reinforcement improves and refines athletes' concentration skills and thereby helps their coping with anxiety and stress.

Self-regulation is useful for athletes because it facilitates their attentional narrowing and focusing. To perform at their best level, athletes must be able to narrow their attention to task relevant cues and ignore irrelevant and disruptive cues in the environment. Easterbrook's [15] cue utilization hypothesis suggests that increases in arousal (or anxiety) produced by internal or external stressors progressively narrow one's attention and create a source of distraction. Landers [16] has extended this hypothesis by proposing that an optimal level of arousal is needed for the maximal athletic performance because attendance to task relevant cues is then at its best. Accordingly, at low levels of arousal, athletes pay too much attention to such irrelevant and disruptive factors as spectators' and other performers' behaviors. As arousal increases to an optimal level, attention is focused on task relevant cues only and irrelevant ones are eliminated, thereby resulting in the maximal performance. On the other hand, if performance anxiety becomes too high and goes beyond the optimal level, the perceptual range narrows so much that valuable task-relevant cues are eliminated; the end result is poor performance. For example, a golfer whose performance anxiety is very low skips his preshot routine and just hits the ball, whereas a golfer who is extremely aroused is not able to narrow his or her attention to task relevant cues such as key swing thoughts or alignment. Instead she or he rushes the shot so as to 'get it over with'. This happens frequently even with world-class golfers who feel 'intimidated' by other performers (e.g. Jack Nicklaus' presence) or circumstances (e.g. to hit the ball over the water to an island green).

It is important to note, however, that there are task and individual differences that mediate this relationship between arousal and performance. Oxendine [17] suggested that the inverted-U relationship between anxiety and performance depends on task complexity:

(1) A high level of arousal is essential for optimal performance in

gross motor activities involving strength, endurance and speed (e.g. weight lifting and sprinting).

(2) A high level of arousal interferes with performance involving complex skills, fine muscle movement, coordination, steadiness, and general concentration (e.g. golf and bowling).

(3) A slightly-above-average level of arousal is preferable to a normal or subnormal state for all motor tasks.

Whether those generalizations have empirical support remains to be shown [18]. It is possible that such a general classification of motor activities is overly simplistic and crude. For example, according to Oxendine, 100- and 200-meter sprinters should develop a high level of arousal before their performance. Yet, such performance anxiety is likely to create excessive tension and tightening of muscles and thereby hinder rather than improve performance. Similarly, it is quite simplistic to assume that activities such as golf only represent fine motor skills. In fact, it has been established that putting (fine motor skill) constitutes about 45% of the total score in golf; in other words, 55% of the total golf performance is gross motor activity. Nevertheless, there is no question about the fact that task or activity differences moderate the arousal-performance relationship. It is just that Oxendine's classification may be an oversimplification.

Another factor related to task differences has to do with the effects of preperformance anxiety on the final outcome. That is, in some sports it is possible to recover from the detrimental effects of excessive preperformance arousal, while in others it is not. For example, a 100-meter sprinter's performance may be fatally impaired by too high a level of arousal. On the other hand, a golfer has about 70 shots left after the first drive and 17 holes after the first hole. So, even if the golfer bogeys the first hole because of the preperformance anxiety and the resultant bad shots, she or he has plenty of chances to 'cool down' and recover. Raymond Floyd, one of the best golfers in the world today, said that every time he steps to the first tee he feels 'butterflies in his stomach', but after the first shot the 'butterflies' are gone and anxiety is reduced to an optimal level. Consistent with this statement, Mahoney and Meyers [19] argued that skilled athletes:

(a) Tend to view their anxiety as, at worst, a nuisance and, at best, an ally in their performance.

(b) Tend to 'pace' their precompetition anxiety more effectively.

(c) Are less focused on their anxiety and more focused on momentary task demands during their performance.

If skilled or veteran athletes can deal more effectively with anxiety than less skilled athletes, it may reflect individual and personality differences between them. It seems that some athletes 'rise to the occasion' and perform better under high pressure situations than others. Those who are highly anxious individuals in general (high on trait anxiety) tend to perform poorly in pressure situations when compared to individuals who are relatively low on trait anxiety. While both high and low trait-anxious athletes appear to exhibit the inverted-U curve between arousal and performance, they differ in the location of the arousal continuum where the inverted-U takes place [20]. That is, high trait anxious athletes' inverted-U is located on the higher end of the arousal continuum and that of low trait-anxious athletes on the lower end of it. This seems to suggest that both types of athletes' maximal performance occurs at the personally optimal level of anxiety, but that level is considerably different for the two groups.

Does this, then, mean that one must have been born with personality to tolerate high pressure situations? Not necessarily. Although it is possible that top-level athletes have gotten so far because of the self-selection process (i.e. highly anxious athletes are weeded out as the competitive level gets tougher), it is also possible that initially high trait-anxious athletes *learn* to control anxiety through their extensive experience of athletic competition or via certain training methods.

Cognitive-Affective Stress Management

It is important to emphasize that a high level of arousal does not necessarily mean high anxiety nor does a low level of arousal necessarily mean relaxation [21]. High arousal, if under personal control and correctly interpreted, can lead to excitement rather than debilitating performance anxiety. Conversely, low arousal can lead to boredom rather than relaxation. Experience of arousal is, therefore, largely an individual matter and must be managed on the individual basis. An optimal level of arousal means that anxiety is at an appropriate and stimulating level for an athlete; it makes him/her excited rather than fearful about his upcoming performance. While common sense suggests that with athletes in general, a bigger problem is too much anxiety rather than too little of it, one cannot go overboard in reducing excessive anxiety. Again, the goal of stress and anxiety management techniques is arousal excitement, not arousal anxiety or arousal boredom.

In general, stress and anxiety management techniques can be considered under an overall title of cognitive-affective training [22]. Although many different techniques have been developed, they all deal with an individual's cognitions and affect. In the presence of cognitive stress or anxiety reactions, athletes' concentration is distracted and their attention directed at task-irrelevant factors. Examples of cognitions that interfere with athletic performance are negative thoughts such as: 'I am not good enough for these guys', 'I cannot afford one more mistake', 'The way I am performing I will have no chance of being among the top ten'. In the presence of affective stress or anxiety reactions, athletes experience extreme autonomic arousal and such physiological reactions as stomach cramps and inability to sleep and rest. Other physiological or physical reactions may include muscular tightness and motor coordination problems.

Cognitive Stress Responses

To combat cognitive and affective stress and anxiety reactions, several approaches can be used. First, whenever possible, stress-causing factors or cues should be removed. As noted earlier, athletes who have been trained in self-instructional and self-monitoring skills are better able to focus their attention on task demands and thereby eliminate distractive external factors. Employment of a little notebook with instructional sheets for self-monitoring procedures can be useful not only for mentally rehearsing certain components of the upcoming performance but also for taking one's attention away from stress-causing cues. In many sports, observing other competitors' performance while awaiting one's turn can become a significant source of preperformance stress and anxiety. For example, think of gymnastics, figure skating and golfing.

Another sport is ski jumping. When this author was competing in ski jumping in Finland at the national level in his early days, it was common that jumpers were watching, while up in the tower, other competitors' jumps. Needless to say, simply watching and waiting for your turn to go down a 90-meter hill was anxiety-producing, and it did not help if other competitors' preceding jumps were bad! At the time, coaches did not know anything about sport psychology nor did the jumpers seem to have any intuitive understanding of self-instruction and self-monitoring processes. Rather than watching others, it would have been much more useful to focus on mentally rehearsing one's performance techniques in various phases of the jump and visualizing the flight. A little notebook containing all the important self-instructions would have helped in preparation for a jump. It is only more recently that such self-monitoring techniques have been used systematically to remove preperformance anxiety and stress. Other simple techniques for removing external stressors include turning one's head away from stress-causing cues, counting trees, examining cloud formations, etc.

If negative thoughts dominate as stress responses, several self-management techniques can be used depending on the fit for a specific athlete. One of them is Meichenbaum's [23] stress inoculation training. This program emphasizes cognitive restructuring and positive self-statements. The basic idea is to first make athletes understand conceptually their response to stressful events and then rehearse various coping techniques; these include positive self-statements. Finally, individuals apply and practice their coping skills and techniques in simulated or real life situations. In golf, for example, because of preperformance anxiety, it is not uncommon that athletes rush their performance so as to 'get it over with'. They think that they are holding others up and therefore feel others are becoming irritated. Such negative thoughts block their attempts to adequately prepare for each shot. Cognitive restructuring is needed in that situation and would mean that the rationality of the thoughts has to be examined carefully. Athletes with such thoughts would be forced to cognitively analyze the situation and reasons for their thinking in that way. They would have to reevaluate their rights as competitors. Negative thoughts would be replaced by positive ones emphasizing their rights to take as much time as others in preparing for each shot.

Replacement of negative thoughts by positive ones should be augmented by positive self-statements and self-talk [24]. However, self-talk is usually negative and nondirectional in nature: 'That is a stupid shot, idiot.' Such statements are emotional and therefore don't help one's concentration. They are typically directed at others and suggest that the person does not normally make such 'stupid' shots. Thus, the person is more concerned about his/her interpersonal image and esteem rather finding remedies for the unsuccessful performance. Such statements may reflect a person's psychological insecurity and lack of self-confidence. It has been shown that successful olympic athletes use performance errors as pieces of information to improve their subsequent performance, whereas the unsuccessful ones tend to react emotionally to their errors [25]. Suinn [26] has used his 'visual motor behavior rehearsal' technique to help athletes rehearse the skill of immediately recovering from errors and refocusing on the ensuing correct responses.

As discussed earlier, athletes have to engage in self-analysis of their performance so as to understand what is going right and wrong. Self-analysis helps athletes detect errors and what to do to correct them. Such an analysis generates directional self-instructions and positive self-statements. For example, if a basketball player charts components of his or her performance and discovers that he or she does relatively poorly on foul shots, he or she should focus on finding key thoughts and visualizing each shot. While preparing for a shot, the player would visualize him/herself jumping, releasing the ball, and the ball flying into the basket. He or she would make a self-instructional correction by saying to him/herself: 'Don't rush the shot. Extend your wrist when releasing the ball. Look at the front rim.' This kind of self-analysis and self-correction would pre-empt negative self-talk and would enhance concentration. The end result would be removal of sources of stress and stress responses. Attentional refocusing is a good technique for controlling arousal, anxiety, and stress.

Affective Stress Responses

In addition to combating cognitive stress responses, athletes' affective stress reactions have to be dealt with. As noted earlier, stressors can lead to excessive heart rate and other symptoms of heightened arousal. They can also result in muscular tightness, restlessness, and problems in motor coordination. Perhaps the most common treatment applied to these stress responses has been Jacobson's [27] progressive relaxation technique or some variations of it. According to Jacobson, one must be able to distinguish between tension and relaxation in order to relax. The technique, therefore, aims at teaching individuals to progressively tense and relax major muscle groups. Similar to this, Wolpe's [28] systematic desensitization technique emphasizes progressive relaxation, although it involves the use of a hierarchy of anxiety-producing stimuli and attempts to master each increasingly more stressful situation. Deep breathing is frequently used to facilitate relaxation and the command 'relax' is supposed to coincide with the exhalation phase. More specific information about breathing and progressive relaxation exercises for athletes can be found in Harris [29].

The advantage of this kind of technique is that no trainers are needed. Athletes can practice it individually and should do it on a daily basis. Sooner or later, it will lead to a coping response that can be readily utilized in stressful situations without interrupting athletic performance. Another simple technique for dealing with affective stress reactions that appear as motor coordination, tightness, and restlessness problems is for athletes to engage in opposite motor behaviors. Thus, athletes would slow down their pace of walking and their movements in general. Rather than making quick and jerky movements they would try to do the opposite and make smooth and wide-ranging motions.

A more complex technique is a psychotherapeutic procedure known as 'induced affect' [30]. Accordingly, individuals are artificially made to experience a high level of anxiety and then taught to bring it under control by coping skills and responses. Needless to say, the technique cannot be used before people have learned the coping responses adequately enough to control the heightened arousal. A high level of arousal is achieved by asking a person to imagine a stressful situation. An example would be a soccer player who faces a penalty kick with one minute left and the game is tied one-to-one. The person is asked to feel the stressfulness of the situation and whilst doing so is told that the feeling is getting stronger and stronger. This is continued until the person responds with considerable anxiety arousal. When the desired level of arousal is achieved, the person is asked to eliminate it by the learned coping skills. The 'turning off' begins by relaxation and is later followed by cognitive self-statements. Smith and Ascough [31] have applied the technique to athletic situations and have combined relaxation and self-statements into the 'integrated coping response'. They have tied this coping response into the breathing cycle so that the athlete makes task-oriented self-statements in the inhalation phase (e.g. 'concentrate on the extension of the left arm') and self-instructions to relax in the exhalation phase.

It is clear that this technique requires considerable training under a professional trainer's supervision before self-regulation can be trusted and accepted. If the lengthy training is a disadvantage, a major advantage is that a person acquires an important coping skill to deal with stress. The person learns to control emotional arousal in various stressful situations. An increased sense of control over stressful stimuli transfers from one situation to another and thereby improves one's overall self-confidence. If performance enhancement does not materialize immediately, it is likely to happen in the long run. At the minimum, an athlete feels better about him/herself, which will be beneficial in the future.

Other Techniques

Besides the techniques covered above there are other methods of mental training that can be used for stress and anxiety management. They include meditation, autogenic training, imagery or visualization, and self-hypnosis. One of the better known meditation techniques is Benson's [32] 'relaxation response' method. Accordingly, a person sits in a quiet environment in a comfortable position with closed eyes and uses a mental device (e.g. the word 'one') to focus attention on something nonarousing. A passive, 'let-it-happen' attitude is emphasized so that thoughts can move freely through consciousness. Mind wandering is controlled by directing attention to the chosen mental device. The technique should be practiced for about 20 min once or twice a day. While the technique cannot be used directly in competitive athletic situations, it can be employed before competition and during the half-time break. Athletes should practice the technique regularly because it helps them achieve a sense of deep relaxation. It also improves their ability to concentrate and discipline the mind.

Autogenic training, a form of meditation and self-hypnosis, is a more involving procedure which requires several months to master the necessary skills. It is based upon the idea of producing two physical sensations, warmth and heaviness and feeling these sensations [33]. Training consists of six stages [29] each of which has to be mastered before moving to the next. In the first stage, a person practices feeling heavy in his/her arms and legs, each at a time and finally together, saying: 'My right arm is heavy', etc. The same format is followed in the second stage, except that a person is trying to feel a warmth sensation in his/her limbs. In the third stage, mental exercises aim at regulating the heartbeat: 'My heartbeat is regular and calm'. The fourth stage focuses on controlling the breathing rate as slow, calm, and relaxed. In the fifth stage, a person strives to feel a sense of warmth in the solar plexis and finally in the sixth stage, a sensation of coolness of the forehead is sought. Some athletes may be able to generate these feelings relatively quickly, while for others the sensations may require extensive training, several times daily for several weeks. When athletes master all the six stages, they can do the entire series in a few minutes. This level of mastery helps them attain a state of relaxation quite readily, and they can then proceed to use imagery for a sense of deeper relaxation.

Imagery is another technique that can be used for stress and anxiety management and performance enhancement. It can be used for many different purposes, from learning and practicing sport skills to controlling physiological responses. In the context of stress and anxiety management, imagery can help in two ways: (a) by producing an optimal level of arousal and relaxation, and (b) by enhancing concentration. Since imagery involves using all the senses to recreate experiences and create new events [34], it can be invoked to control such physiological responses as heart rate, respiration, blood pressure, and skin temperature. The benefit of this is obvious in many sports like biathlon in which athletes have to stop to shoot a target with their rifle after several kilometers of strenuous cross-country skiing. Similarly, imagery can be employed to control arousal stress and anxiety before an execution of athletic movements. Imagery can also help by enhancing athletes' ability to concentrate. Jack Nicklaus is a classic example of an athlete who has used imagery to improve his concentration and enhance performance. Before each shot, he visualizes the ball in the target, the ball's flight to the target, and his execution of the swing to get the ball to the target.

Imagery involves use of visual, auditory, olfactory, tactile, and kinesthetic senses to recreate experiences or to create new experiences. Images can be created by using any one of these senses separately or altogether. Vealey [34] argues that using all the appropriate senses helps athletes create more vivid images and that the more vivid images lead to a greater effect on performance. Most frequently, however, imagery is thought of in terms of visual images produced by memory. This can happen by observing others or oneself perform a certain skill and then using such a mental picture as a basis of one's performance. Or, visual imagery can be used to prepare for future performance like the Swedish National golf team did in 1990. For months ahead of the World Amateur Golf Championship tournament in New Zealand, Swedes sent a person to take pictures of all the 18 holes, so that the team members could visualize themselves playing each hole. By the time the team arrived at the tournament site, they were well acquainted with each hole and all the potential problems. The team shocked the golfing world not only by winning but by lapping the field.

Scientific evidence for imagery is strong [35]. Positive effects of imagery have been documented in many different sports, from basketball free-throw shooting and tennis serving to muscular endurance tasks and alpine skiing. If positive imagery does not always improve performance over the baseline (without imagery), it at least prevents a degradation of performance by negative imagery [36]. The literature also suggests that mental rehearsal of task performance coupled with mental depiction of performance outcome is more effective in enhancing motor skill performance than imagery involving only mental rehearsal. So, golfers, for example, should imagine not only the putting stroke but also the ball going in the hole. There is also evidence that combined with other mental training techniques, imagery has positive effects. Kendall et al. [37] reported that an imagery rehearsal along with relaxation and self-talk constituted an effective treatment package that enhanced the performance of specific defensive basketball skill during the actual competition in the intercollegiate basketball games.

It is important to stress, however, that imagery is a skill like any other physical skill in sports. An athlete has to believe in it and has to practice it regularly. Basic training consists of three sets of imagery exercises planned to (1) develop athletes' visual images; (2) to control their images, and (3) to increase their self-perceptions of their sport performance. Specific exercises for these components of imagery can be found in Vealey [34] and Porter and Foster [38].

Finally, self-hypnosis as a mental training technique should be mentioned. Self-hypnosis represents 'inner mental training' and is used in combination with other programs of mental practice (39). Its objective is to increase the individual's ability to concentrate and to mentally relax when needed. Emphasis in training is placed on increased self-control. Athletes are taught to use triggers to induce enhanced relaxation and concentration. Hypnosis is a state of mind, an alternative state of consciousness often more popularly referred to by athletes as 'zone', 'hot night', 'being in the tunnel', 'flow', etc. While attainment of such an ideal state of mind cannot be guaranteed, the self-hypnotic state increases one's chances of achieving it or getting close to it. To this extent, triggers are effective means of inducing self-hypnosis and can be learned through a systematic training with a professional.

Unestahl [39] described the effect in one bowler: 'When I stick my fingers into the ball (his trigger), I can notice the lights in the room go down. After some seconds there exists only one light corridor, which is my own alley with the marks and the pins. This lasts until the ball hits the pins. Then the light comes back and I become aware of what's happening on the other alleys. This gives me a very good feeling of control. I can relax and rest between my hits because I know that as soon as I stick my fingers into the ball, the total concentration will be there.' To achieve this level of control over self-hypnotic states requires several weeks' training with a professional. But every athlete is capable of learning self-hypnosis as a natural alternative state of mind or consciousness. As Unestahl [39] states, the effects of inner mental training increase with training and are clearest and most evident after a long, regular training period.

It is important to emphasize that the psychoregulatory techniques discussed above should be used in conjunction with other training methods, such as a proper diet, physiotheraphy, and massage. It should also be kept in mind that mental training is no substitute for physical training. Outstanding athletic performance requires both. Also, the following prerequisites must be met before psychoregulatory techniques can be successfully applied [33]:

(1) Athletes must participate in the program actively and voluntarily from the beginning. In the absence of a positive attitude toward the psychoregulatory training (PRT), it will be difficult for the athlete to apply the technique successfully.

(2) The PRT should be applied over a long period of time in training, especially in those stages where training is the most intensive. It is important that PRT be effective and that it be perceived as such by the athlete.

(3) It is recommended that PRTs not be used until the procedure has been mastered. Again, the importance of maintaining a positive attitude in the athlete cannot be overestimated, and a necessary condition of maintaining a positive attitude is that the PRT not be applied carelessly or in a haphazard manner.

Summary and Conclusions

This paper has examined mental training and its role in athletic performance. In general, mental training refers to skill training for performance enhancement and emphasizes self-regulation of sport performance. It strives to improve athletes' cognitive and affective skills so as to better their performance. The process of self-regulation stresses the importance of goal-setting and positive expectations for success, self-monitoring relevant behaviors, self-evaluation of performance against standards, and self-reinforcement or self-punishment.

Research suggests that athletes should be directed to set their goals personally, their goals should be specific and difficult but attainable, and the overall goal should be broken down into 'proximal sub-goals'. Athletes should learn to self-monitor their performance because self-monitoring promotes the use of highly specific, nonemotional feedback and facilitates accurate self-evaluation. Self-monitoring also facilitates attentional focusing and encourages the use of self-instructions. Athletes who engage in the self-regulation process through self-monitoring, self-evaluation, and self-reinforcement protect themselves from coaches' repeated negative feedback as well.

One of the main aspects of mental training is anxiety and stress management. Athletes must learn to handle and regulate their anxiety and stress, so that they both can be brought under control and to the optimal level. To this extent, the self-regulation process improves and refines athletes' concentration skills and thereby helps their coping with anxiety and stress. There is considerable evidence in the literature to suggest that an optimal level of arousal is needed for the maximal athletic performance because attendance to task relevant cues is then at its best. There are, however, task and individual differences that mediate this relationship between arousal and performance. For example, those who are highly anxious individuals in general tend to perform poorly in pressure situations when compared to individuals who are relatively low on trait anxiety.

In general, stress and anxiety management techniques can be combined under an overall title of cognitive-affective training. In the presence of cognitive stress or anxiety reactions, athletes' concentration is distracted and their attention directed at task-irrelevant factors. Employment of little notebooks with instructional sheets for self-monitoring procedures can be useful not only for mentally rehearsing certain components of the upcoming performance but also for taking one's attention away from stress-causing cues. Of several self-management techniques, stress inoculation training is useful with its emphasis on cognitive restructuring and positive self-statements. Replacement of negative thoughts by positive ones should be augmented by positive self-statements and self-talk. When athletes engage in self-analysis of their performance so as to understand what is going right or wrong, they are able to detect errors and what to do to correct them. Such an analysis generates directional self-instructions and positive self-statements.

In addition to cognitive stress responses, athletes' affective reactions have to be brought under control. Several progressive relaxation techniques exist and aim at teaching individuals to progressively tense and relax major muscle groups. Others involve the use of a hierarchy of anxiety-producing stimuli and attempts to master each increasingly more stressful situation. In the 'induced affect' method, individuals are artificially made to experience a high level of anxiety and then are taught to bring it under control by coping skills and responses. Other methods of mental training that can be used for stress and anxiety management include meditation, autogenic training, imagery, and self-hypnosis. Of these, imagery has become very popular among athletes. It involves using all senses to recreate experiences and create new events. The literature suggests that mental rehearsal of task performance coupled with mental depiction of performance outcome is more effective in enhancing motor skill performance than imagery involving only mental rehearsal. Research also supports the idea that an imagery rehearsal along with relaxation and self-talk constitutes an effective treatment package that enhances performance.

It is important to emphasize that the use of any psychoregulatory techniques requires that athletes believe in them, apply them in training over a long period of time, and master them technically and procedurally. A positive attitude toward mental training in general and toward specific techniques in particular is a necessary condition for performance enhancement. Athletes who are mentally strong are able to learn from mistakes and failures rather than react to them negatively, they maintain positive attitude throughout, and they know how to handle stress and anxiety correctly.

References

1   Iso-Ahola SE, Hatfield B: Psychology of Sports: A Social Psychological Approach. Dubuque, Brown, 1986, pp 157, 182.
2   Williams JM: Integrating and implementing a psychological skills training program; in Williams JM (ed.): Applied Sport Psychology. Palo Alto, Mayfield, 1986, pp 301–324.
3   Mahoney MJ: Sport Psychology. AG Stanley Hall Lecture. Atlanta, American Psychological Association, 1988.
4   Kirschenbaum DS: Self-regulation of sport performance. Med. Sci. Sports Exerc 1987;19:S106–S113.
5   Feltz DL, Landers DM: The effects of mental practice on motor skill learning and performance: A meta-analysis. J Sport Psychol 1983;5:25–57.
6   Morgan WP: Test of champions: The iceberg profile. Psychol Today 1980;14(July):92–102, 108.
7   Bandura A, Schunk DH: Cultivating competence, self-efficacy, and intrinsic interest through proximal self-evaluation. J Personal Social Psychol 1981;41:586–598.
8   Locke EA, Shaw KN, Saari LM, Latham GP: Goal setting and task performance: 1969–1980. Psychol Bull 1981;90:125–152.
9   Iso-Ahola SE, Mobily K: Psychological momentum: A phenomenon and its empirical (unobtrusive) validation in competitive sport tournament. Psychol Rep 1980;46:391–401.
10 Iso-Ahola SE, Blanchard WJ: Psychological momentum and competitive sports: A field study. Perceptual Mot Skills 1986;62:763–768.

11   Cummings LL, Schwab DP, Rosen M: Performance and knowledge of results as
     determinants of goal setting. J Appl Psychol 1971;55:526–530.
12   Jones SL, Nation JR, Massad P: Immunizing against learned helplessness in man. J
     Abnorm Psychol 1977;86:75–83.
13   Smith RE, Smoll FL, Curtis B: Coach effectiveness training: A cognitive-behavioral
     approach to enhancing relationship skills in youth sport coaches. J Sport Psychol
     1979;1:59–75.
14   Kirschenbaum DS, Smith RJ: Sequencing effects in simulated coach feedback: Continu-
     ous criticism, or praise, can debilitate performance. J Sport Psychol 1983;5:332–342.
15   Easterbrook JA: The effect of emotion on cue utilization and the organization of
     behavior. Psychol Rev 1959;66:183–201.
16   Landers DM: The arousal-performance relationship revisited. Res Q 1980;51:77–90.
17   Oxendine J: Emotional arousal and motor performance. Quest 1970;13:23–32.
18   Hackfort D, Spielberger CD (eds): Anxiety in Sports: An International Perspective.
     Washington, Hemisphere, 1989.
19   Mahoney MJ, Meyers AW: Anxiety and athletic performance: Traditional and cogni-
     tive-developmental perspectives; in Hackfort D, Spielberger CD (eds): Anxiety in
     Sports. Washington, Hemisphere, 1989, pp 77–94.
20   Klavora P: An attempt to derive inverted-U curves based on the relationship between
     anxiety and athletic performance; in Landers DM, Christina RW (eds): Psychology of
     Motor Behavior and Sport. Champaign, Human Kinetics, 1978.
21   Kerr JH: Anxiety, arousal, and sport performance: An application of reversal theory; in
     Hackfort D, Spielberger CD (eds): Anxiety in Sports. Washington, Hemisphere, 1989,
     pp 137–151.
22   Crocker PRE, Alderman RB, Smith FMR: Cognitive-affective stress management
     training with high performance youth volleyball players: Effects on affect, cognition, and
     performance. J Sport Exerc Psychol 1988;10:448–460.
23   Meichenbaum D: Cognitive Behavior Modification: An Integrative Approach. New
     York, Plenum Press, 1977.
24   Bunker L, Williams JM: Cognitive techniques for improving performance and building
     confidence; in Williams J (ed): Applied Sport Psychology. Palo Alto, Mayfield, 1986, pp
     235–255.
25   Mahoney MJ, Avener M: Psychology of the elite athlete: An exploratory study. Cogn
     Ther Res 1977;1:135–141.
26   Suinn RM (ed): Psychology in Sports: Methods and Applications. Minneapolis,
     Burgess, 1980.
27   Jacobson E: Progressive Relaxation. Chicago, University of Chicago Press, 1938.
28   Wolpe J: The Practice of Behavior Therapy. New York, Pergamon Press, 1969.
29   Harris DV: Relaxation and energizing techniques for regulation of arousal; in Williams
     JM (ed): Applied Sport Psychology. Palo Alto, Mayfield, 1986, pp 185–207.
30   Sipprelle CN: Induced anxiety. Psychotherapy 1967;4:36–40.
31   Smith RE, Ascough JC: Induced affect in stress management training; in Burchfield S
     (ed): Stress: Psychological and Physiological Interactions. Washington, Hemisphere,
     1985.
32   Benson H: The Relaxation Response. New York, Avon Books, 1975.
33   Schellenberger H: Psychology of Team Sports. Toronto, Sport Books, 1990.
34   Vealey RS: Imagery training for performance enhancement; in Williams JM (ed):
     Applied Sport Psychology. Palo Alto, Mayfield, 1986, pp 209–231.
35   Lee L: Psyching up for a muscular endurance task: Effects of image content on
     performance and mood state. J Sport Exerc Psychol 1990;12:66–73.

36   Woolfolk RL, Parrish MW, Murphy SM: The effects of positive and negative imagery on motor skill performance. Cogn Ther Res 1985;9:335–341.

37   Kendall G, Hrycaiko D, Martin GL, Kendall T: The effects of an imagery rehearsal, relaxation, and self-talk package on basketball game performance. J Sport Exerc Psychol 1990;12:157–166.

38   Porter K, Foster J: Visual Athletics: Visualizations for Peak Sports Performance. Dubuque, Brown, 1990.

39   Unestahl L-E: Self-hypnosis; in Williams JM (ed): Applied Sport Psychology. Palo Alto, Mayfield, 1986, pp 285–300.

Dr. Seppo E. Iso-Ahola, PhD, 2367 HLHP Building, College of Health and Human Performance, University of Maryland, College Park, MD 20742 (USA)

Subject Index